Getting Back in the River

The GBU Letters

Beginning Life Anew

by
Sara Dumaine Brouillet, Ph.D.

Beginning Life Anew

Neither this book nor any other can replace the services of a qualified health professional. Please use the contents and suggestions herein, as appropriate, to help in communicating with your physician, therapist, clergy, friend.

Unless otherwise specifically stated, the names and identifying characteristics of all persons in this book have been changed.

Father's Press, LLC
Lee's Summit, MO
816.600.6288
www.fatherspress.com

Cover & drawings in watercolor by Martha Reid Hudson.

Cover design by Diane Landskroener.

Illustrations by Penelope Kay Hollingsworth.

Digital Imaging by The Finishing Touch.

Book design by Sara Dumaine Brouillet.

Beginning Life Anew

From the river to the sea
...And when you emerge from the sea of silence...

Those whom God calls into his silence will enter a vortex
which will shatter them into little pieces. Looking here and
there you will see fragments of a human being.
You will behold your own fragmentation and wonder
why you do not die. I do not know why. God knows.
But in his silence he will gather together your fragments. And
when you emerge from the sea of silence
you will become like thunder, thunder that passes beyond
the galaxies as if it were a bird sent forth
to preach the Gospel to the whole universe.

Catherine Doherty, <u>Molchanie</u>, 2001

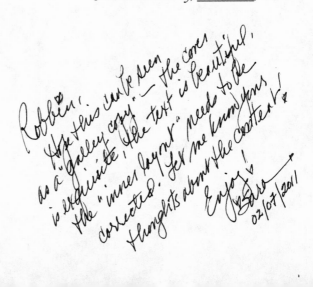

Beginning Life Anew

Dedication

For Anna, Maggie, and Sam

With love and thankfulness to my entire family: especially, my parents for their love, depth of truth, and goodness of mind in serving others; to Rebecca and Bill, and George and Stevie, for modeling loving relationships. There are so many others to thank, not named, all of whom know in their hearts our unending personal and professional friendship; and, especially, Robbin, Martha, Do, Mary, Cynthia, Mark, John, Shea, Sian, Chuck and Lorna, Hamp and Elizabeth, Bill and Elizabeth, Carmella, Tom, Bill, Maureen, Laura, Bob, Diane, Penny, Ralph, Dan, Flo, Faith, and Grace. To Mike Smitley who follows the Lord's guidance in all aspects of his publishing work: with gratefulness for Mike's healing, and for his wise and unending encouragement.

With respect for and thankfulness to each of my clients for perseverance in doing their work to stay in a well direction, yielding to grace.

With love and thankfulness to Martha Reid Hudson, 88 years young, whose glorious gifts in watercolor reflect her discovery of creation in the *depth* of the river, and in the grace and power of feathers; these, being only two aspects of our shared joy in and appreciation of the sacred in light.

With humble thanksgiving to God for the life of *birds* whose wings of strength represent the ability to be uplifted and eternally renewed, whose individual variability is virtually endless, and whose *feathers* ~ in design from the smallest to the largest, function interdependently and in concert with God's exquisite purposes of beauty and transporting life, while literally *being as light as a feather, the breath of the Holy Spirit.*

Beginning Life Anew

CONTENTS

Beginning Life Anew

Chapter One

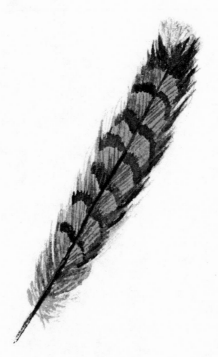

Be still and know that I am God.

Psalm 46:10

Beginning Life Anew

Chapter One

Then he led me back along the bank of the river. As
I went back, I saw upon the bank of the river very
many trees on the one side and on the other. And he
said to me, "This water flows toward the eastern
region and goes down into the Arabah; and when it
enters the stagnant waters of the sea, the water will
become fresh. And wherever the river goes every
living creature which swarms will live, and there will
be very many fish; for this water goes there, that the
waters of the sea may become fresh; so everything
will live where the river goes."[1,2]

We need the waters of the sea to heal us and yield the
creation of new life, and to help us in *getting back in the river*
when we are experiencing the pain of death or significant loss
and little makes sense to us. We need the restorative, buoyant,
able to be salt again, depths of God's unimaginable healing and
love, known to us as relationship with the Word of God made
flesh, Jesus Christ. In seeking to heal their recent loss, a family
asked me, "How do we get there?" It is the quintessentially
exquisite, gentle, yet, persistent and faithful love of the Holy
Spirit that brings healing. Thanks be to God. God's loving
relationship with us in the person of Jesus and in the power of
the Holy Spirit *heals* grief and loss. God says to us, "*Nothing*
can separate us from the love of Christ." The Lord will go to
any length to restore us to God, take anyone and anything, in
order to be first in our hearts and minds, and only then, to bring
us new life in Christ for God's eternal purpose. The love of God
offers grace to heal in a moment; yet, for most of us, grieving is
a process known as bereavement that moves through many
months, often years, especially when we are doing little to
embrace our healing.

The purpose of this book is to offer actual steps of *core healing* in bereavement: the writing of two letters, one quite distinct from the other. Each letter is both an action we can choose to take and a process within us in healing loss. Why read a book about grieving when others are writing about seemingly more joyous avenues of relationship with God? Joy is within and of God, and known to us in the Lord's blessed actions in healing the loss. Most of us have heard the phrase, "Time heals all wounds." Are we not supposed to *just wait* until an undefined amount of time has passed and the loss, somewhat magically, will have gone away? If we do nothing, it is improbable that time will heal our deep pain and sadness. When we seek the Lord, the Logos, the Word of God, and are open to the Holy Spirit's promptings, the quiet voice within, God will guide our healing as we humbly and thankfully continue to seek and to follow. We may be a member of or visit a parish community, join a prayer group, hold a Bible study, actively participate in a sacred texts book club, share with friends and family our journey with God, be on a quiet walk in the woods or by the water, go on spiritual retreats or attend workshops to help us heal, and read recommended writings, prayers, books, and articles. God uses everything and, like the lost sheep, not one of us will perish whether or not we see God's abiding grace.

This book offers actual steps to genuine and deep healing of significant loss. Getting Back in the River tenders beneficence in that: 1) the inspired word and work of God created the writing and contents of this book; and, 2) the GBU letters work to heal grief and loss. The impetus to write the initial GBU letters began for me 21 years ago, right in the middle, the fifth, of nine deaths. The GBU letters (*good, bad,* and *uglies*) contain your true thoughts and feelings about the loss, those of which you are conscious and those of which you may be unaware. The letters help to bring to conscious awareness formerly hidden thoughts and feelings. God is faithful: *to see ourselves as the Lord sees us and, hopefully, as in grace we yield ourselves to become more like Jesus, the Christ of God,* is to recognize and acknowledge that love heals and is one of innumerable, often numinous gifts from God. God *is* love and love is *of* God; there

4

are no two ways about this. The truth: only the love of God creates new life.

No matter the loss or how it occurred, writing the GBU letters yields deep healing. Along the way, you will understand a process called *secondary gain* which is the unconscious benefit to be derived from holding on to your loss. When you choose to write the GBU letters, you shall *know* love, which is *of* God, sacred, eternal, and lives forever. It is the experience of over 2,000 people who have written these letters that the Holy Spirit brings healing gifts of sacred relationship with the loving spirit of those for whom they were grieving. The gifts of God do not stop; rather, they continue, humble us in their depth, surprise and delight in drawing us closer to God and to God's blessing as we are given to understand a higher purpose in the loss which otherwise may remain obscure or unknown. At the very least, you can experience forgiveness of and from self, other, God.

You can be brave, risk that you shall laugh again, be in life again, and find yourself *getting back in the river*. Or, you may hold on to the apathy, anger, sadness or despair, protecting your loss from the light, from its gift. The choice is yours. I hope you choose to begin life anew.

Grieving: What Is It?

People in sorrow, from whatever cause, tend to follow a pattern that includes multiple stages. Dr. Erich Lindemann, a former Harvard University professor, first described the grief process in the American Journal of Psychiatry. Lindemann discusses the difference between normal grief response and morbid or abnormal grief reactions. The key in any type of grieving is to help ourselves accept the struggle of working through our grief. In Lindemann's terms, the individual has to be helped to "extricate himself from the bondage to the deceased and find new patterns of rewarding interaction."[3] Lindemann notes five markers of acute grief: 1) somatic distress (of or relating to the body); 2) preoccupation with the image of the deceased; 3) guilt; 4) hostile reactions; and, 5) loss of patterns of conduct.[4] The key is to help the grieving person face the loss by wrestling openly with it. When *we* do so, we come through the grieving experience stronger, with a deeper understanding of ourselves and of our relationship with God, often gaining insight about the meaning of the loss in our lives. We are able to support others, too, as they work through their grieving. We are newly anchored in how *love* lives and behaves, in what forgiveness means, and in depths of sacred relationship with one another.

Dr. Elisabeth Kübler-Ross identified five stages in the grief process in her book, <u>On Death and Dying</u>: 1) denial; 2) anger; 3) bargaining; 4) depression; and, 5) acceptance.[5] Kübler-Ross described her process of experientially becoming attuned to the reality of her own death as she related to dying patients, a process in Gestalt psychology known as *congruence*. Often, death is seen, felt, and spoken about as something alien to and *out of sync* with life when, in fact, it is very much a part of everyday living. Spiritually, these processes are a part of *dying to self*, a phrase first attributed to William Law, a 17th Century theologian.[6]

Dying to self is a lifelong process of its own, largely lived out in the first two commandments, calling us to love the Sacred, God, and the sacred in one another. When we consider the depth of sacred love, holiness, within what we may call the heart of God to us, or even *ponder* what we know to be unspeakably deep human love which also is of God, the light given is incisive, pure, the barest refraction of the source, and, yet, full, true, and eternal. We are called in the first commandment: "You shall love the Lord your God with all your heart, and with all your soul, and with all your mind;" and, in the second: "You shall love your neighbor as yourself."[7] We are called by God in Christ Jesus: "This is my commandment, that you love one another as I have loved you."[8] <u>In grace, we are learning and teaching *love* throughout our lives. In truth, most of us stumble miserably in keeping these commandments. When we think we are the closest to *being* this love, we have the farthest to go, still so very much to learn from the quintessential love that is our Lord. Yet, at some point, *infinite* points, we are united with all that is of God, the sacred. In these</u>

moments, we know God's love and faithfulness; these, we are called to give to one another, to *be* with one another. It is ours to seek diligently, and to be humble, joyous, and thankful, abounding in God's prevenient grace and healing.

We know the Holy Spirit empowers us to love and to be faithful as God in Jesus is with us. When we love as we are called to do, when we die to self, then we are living life in the grace and power of the Holy Spirit. At first, we resist our partial understanding of this sacred and profound teaching: we want things to go our way; think of this as our ego-driven self. We do not surrender easily our way for something as "nebulous" as *God*, especially if God has taken someone or something we love. Right here, we are asked to die to our ego self and live in the sacred self, the latter not being a duality, rather the deeper integration of our *be*ing, who God is within us. It is not that we do not want to be with the beloved person or pet or other loss, we do. It is more that God brings healing, restitution to the loving relationship, to know God in its love, drawing us ever closer to God. We are one with the Lord, truer reflections of and in relationship with the resurrected Christ, and with each other.

We, like the people of Judah and the people of Jerusalem, do not obey easily. Each of us has one-to-three major life *learnings* and an untold number of life lessons. We help each other to discern our life lessons as we pray, act lovingly, and walk with one another, forgiving, *in-kind-ness*. Dr. John E. Davis first taught me that our life learnings will come around and around until we complete the work particular to us in that learning.[9] In my own experience and with others, accepting the grace and putting in the effort to complete our part of the learning, takes what looks like a life journey piece and transforms it (and us) to lifelong journey *peace* within. Life is prayer and homework, and we all get a boatload of homework, my clients often hear me say. God is faithful: "And I am sure that he who began a good work in you will bring it to completion at the day of Jesus Christ."[10]

A stable brain which is difficult to sustain without an inner quietness, allows our mind to grasp what the Holy Spirit in our thoughts and emotions is enlightening for us, where we need to learn and to grow, to be well and at-peace in the moment. Once, and it takes some time, the particular life learning becomes an integrated aspect of our sacred self, we rarely, if ever, need to repeat it. We die to our smaller wants to live in blessed and abundant life, one step at a time. Our one-to-three significant life learnings (not our thousands of lessons) are extremely difficult for us. Our life learnings are unique to us, though recognizable to others in the imperative, intrinsic quality of meaningful healing for each person. If we know enough about someone, everything the person does makes sense; *and*, without a life intervention (available and offered constantly in our relationship with God), it is unlikely the person will change, grow, or even adapt to, let alone create a healthier life. Three, universal, life *learnings* are: we cannot make another person do anything (sometimes not ourselves, either), we cannot change the past, and we are not the Savior.[11]

No one surrenders easily, particularly when our surrender includes grappling with the loss of a family member, part of our community, even part of ourselves. It is a lifelong process to discover some compatibility between life and death, even their synchronicity, and our respectful and loving acceptance of their oneness. Learning to live with death as a reality of life helps us to be present, more aware and thankful, and at-peace; it is a task of the psyche which means soul in ancient Greek. Different types of grief may distance us from even considering the surrender of our vulnerable self.

Anticipatory grief defines the process in which we move through all of the stages of grieving in advance of the loss as a form of protection against when the actual loss or loss notification occurs; for example, when an unwell person is diagnosed as terminally ill.

In contrast, acute or sudden grief has an immediate finality about it, the first response being *shock*.

Many reactions may occur at the point of shock:
+ Expressing emotion or not;
+ Feeling depressed and very lonely to the point of physical withdrawal, certainly emotional withdrawal (*the Jell-O pool*, see page 20);

+ Experiencing somatic (body or physical) symptoms of distress;

+ Experiencing panic and/or acute symptoms of anxiety (elevated pulse or heart rate, difficulty breathing, chest tightness or pain), because we cannot think of anything except the loss and we become paralyzed by that fear;

+ Feeling a sense of guilt, even what still could be called neurotic guilt (the latter is a matter of degree and dysfunction);

+ Being filled with deep feelings of anger or resentment;

+ Resisting a return to a more *normal* pace of life (our life as the mourner has changed irrevocably); the grieving, as yet, has not been worked through and we do not know God's gift in the loss; and,

+ Hyper-functioning, as if the sudden loss had not occurred. Hope is an elusive feeling, even construct, because at this place of shock-response we could not begin to think about or affirm a new, healthy, healed, peaceful, and calm reality.

Complicated grief is the existence of multiple sources of loss, simultaneously. Working through one loss at a time requires depth, honesty, perseverance, a certain degree of balance in being alone and with others, the gift of keeping our faith even in surrender, and acknowledgment of our true feelings about the loss, while being kind to ourselves. Grieving one significant loss, itself, can be daunting because healing any significant loss is a multifaceted process. We may feel inconsolable. Healing complicated grief almost always necessitates help from others which is available in a grief support group, working with a bereavement counselor or with a therapist who has grief-support experience. Working with others opens the way for the Holy Spirit to reach us in another's experience of loss or to reach another through our experience. Too easily we forget God's guidance and presence in our healing:

> Yet it was I who taught Ephraim to walk, I took
> them up in my arms; but they did not know that
> I healed them. I led them with cords of compassion,
> with the bands of love, and I became to them as one

9

who eases the yoke on their jaws, and I bent down to them and fed them. [12]

Multi-generational grief incorporates the healing sequences, above, and the need for support. Dual-diagnosis or co-occurring disorders work in the mental health field would suggest application of the term *multi-generational grief* to those in a family system steeped in various forms of unacknowledged or yet-to-be-worked-through addictive behaviors. In her helpful book, After the Tears, Jane Middleton-Moz writes of how, in generation after generation, the painful cycle of subtle, yet, profound, relationship dynamics only begins to improve when the disease process is stopped; examples include alcoholism, gambling, drug abuse or dependence, and pornography. [13]

Multi-generational grief symptoms often seem phantom like:

+ A parent who has not grieved his/her own childhood losses sees the child/ren *primarily* as the way to self-fulfillment, thereby undermining the child's development, and the steps necessary for healthy adult, interpersonal relationships for the parent and the child/ren;

+ Unresolved grief in these families leads to members being emotionally unavailable and isolated, thereby persisting in denial of earlier losses, and to continued use of defense mechanisms such as repression and suppression, to name only two;

+ Deficits in loving attachment include ignoring a child's basic rights to be safe (my use of the phrase *primum non nocere*, first do no harm), to experience trust, to be nurtured, and to learn how to cope with and grow through various disappointments; and,

+ Suppression of guilt may lead to people seeking healthier life elsewhere or "outside."

Remember, ***we will cope at all costs***. The dynamics noted, above, and the need to pursue help in creating healthy family relationships may continue to be denied, such that any person who remains in the system without support and seeks to recover, to be *well*, is hampered in accessing real opportunities for healthy life.

The internal conflict and struggles associated with death and loss can be dangerous in other ways. David Edwards cites Perls, Hefferline, and Goodman, who state, "Mourning as a means of letting go of the old self to change, explains why mourning is attended by self-destructive behaviors like scratching the skin, beating the breast, tearing the hair;" and, we could add, the abuse of medication or involvement in any numbing behavior.[14]

A primary goal of psychotherapy or counseling in the grief process is not to weaken the conflict, but to strengthen the inner self (uniting the ego self and the sacred self) which helps us to evolve as healthy and loving people who work through loss while remaining as present as we can each day. Our arduous inner work yields depth within us; gradually, we become the people God creates for God's purposes. Healing the suffering connected with grief, loss, and separation can produce a measure of growth and beginning life anew not experienced in any other way. Satan challenges the Lord's word that Job (1:16), a "blameless and upright" man, when tested, would not curse God. Job loses everything, all is taken: his children, his home, his property. We learn:

> Then Job arose, and rent his robe, and shaved his head, and fell upon the ground, and worshiped. And he said, "Naked I came from my mother's womb, and naked shall I return; the Lord gave, and the Lord has taken away; blessed be the name of the Lord."
> In all this Job did not sin or charge God with wrong.[15] Job loses his health, not his integrity.[16] Job laments being born, yet does not curse God.[17]

Martin Luther observed:

> A theology of glory calls evil good and good evil. A theology of the cross calls a thing what it actually is. This is clear: He who does not know Christ does not know God hidden in suffering. Therefore he prefers works to suffering, glory to the cross, strength to weakness, wisdom to folly, and, in general, good to evil. These are the people whom the apostle calls "enemies of

the cross of Christ" [Phil. 3:18], for they hate the cross and suffering and love works and the glory of works. Thus they call the good of the cross evil and the evil of a deed good. God can be found only in suffering and the cross, as has already been said. Therefore the friends of the cross say that the cross is good and works are evil, for through the cross works are destroyed and the old Adam, who is especially edified by works, is crucified. It is impossible for a person not to be puffed up by his good works unless he has first been deflated and destroyed by suffering and evil until he knows that he is worthless and that his works are not his but God's.[18]

The purely-mental-health perspective would struggle with any notion of people considering themselves to be worthless. Such understanding is incomplete and focuses upon only our very human nature, and, as Martin Luther remarked, not on whose we are and for whom we live and breathe, created as we are by God and in the image of God, and for God's purpose. The water of baptism joins our life with the resurrected Christ, and it is the indwelling Holy Spirit who empowers us to become who God creates us to be. It is extremely difficult, impossible really, in "our own power" even to *surrender* ourselves; to do so, we need the love of Jesus Christ and the fellowship of the Holy Spirit of God.

Rabbi Harold S. Kushner wrote, "One of the most important things that any religion can teach us is what it means to be human. The Bible's version of Man is as fundamental to its overall outlook as its vision of God. Two passages at the very beginning of the Bible teach us about being human, and tell us how we, as human beings, relate to God and to the world around us."[19] Kushner speaks of the beginning of Genesis, as it is written that we are made in the image of God, and "at the climax of the Creation process, [where] God is represented as saying, 'Let us make Man in our image.' "[20]

When we become *aware* (even minutely) that we cannot carry our own burdens without the Lord, and Jesus invites us to give them all to him, we are at-peace, mentally healthy, and,

in the power of the Holy Spirit, able to share one another's burdens and to walk together no matter what it takes.
Our core healing of loss in Jesus, the Logos, the love and Word of God, the Christ, the Messiah of God, creates openness within us for more abundant life. When asked why he was leaving Harvard University to become a part of the L'Arche Community in Toronto, Canada, Henri Nouwen replied, "Because I want to see what they can teach me."[21]

Water

Getting Back in the River became the title of this book long after the idea of writing it took hold. The symbol of the river or moving water conveys the idea of actively being at-peace, flowing with the sacred and mindful tides of life. A Psalm of David teaches, ". . . the river of God is full of water; thou providest their grain, for so thou hast prepared it. Thou waterest its furrows abundantly, settling its ridges, softening it with showers, and blessing its growth."[22] In Genesis 39:1-23, we read of God's blessing upon Joseph's work as overseer of Potiphar's house and of his generosity with Joseph. Even when imprisoned following an untruth from Potiphar's wife, God continues to bless and affirm Joseph. Of Joseph, Paul Kretzmann writes:

> Thus many an innocent Christian has been obliged to suffer wrongfully, to be suspected and accused of crimes of various kinds. In spite of all that, however, the believers place their trust in the mercy of God. "But the Lord was with Joseph, and showed him mercy, and gave him favor in the sight of the keeper of the prison." The hearts of men are in the hands of the Lord, and he can guide them like rivers of water.[23]

Continuing the citation from Ezekiel on the first page of this chapter, we read:

13

And he said to me, "Son of man, have you seen this?" Then he led me back along the bank of the river. ". . . for this water goes there, that the waters of the sea may become fresh; so everything will live where the river goes. Fisherman will stand beside the sea; from Engedi to Eneglaim it will be a place for the spreading of nets; its fish will be of very many kinds, like the fish of the Great Sea. But its swamps and marshes will not become fresh; they are to be left for salt. And on the banks, on both sides of the river, there will grow all kinds of trees for food. Their leaves will not wither nor their fruit fail, but they will bear fresh fruit every month, because the water for them flows from the sanctuary. Their fruit will be for food, and their leaves for healing."[24]

It is helpful to remember: we are water; it is the most abundant substance of which we are made. Science tells us that we change from being approximately 90 percent water at birth, to being 70 percent to 75 percent water as healthy adults, to being about 50 percent water or less, relatively quickly upon death. Dr. Masaru Emoto, now mainstreamed, has contributed the results of his more than three decades of scientific research on the crystalline structure of water. Dr. Emoto clearly and astonishingly demonstrates: *as* water freezes, progressing from a liquid to a solid state while, simultaneously, the water is exposed to varying words, the very structure of the crystals changes significantly. Emoto's research surprises us in being able to capture the impact of our words "on" water. Given our composition, God with us, and the Word made flesh, it is not a surprise, more a gift of grace-filled understanding that our words, how we speak with one another and our self-statements, have the power to change us. The use of particular words, themselves, and the declension of noun/verb dyads indicate *relationship* in many languages. The Word of God, the Logos, Jesus in our midst, the Christ of our being, signify relationship, and cleanse and teach and heal and sanctify us in the power of the Holy Spirit. Paul speaks to the Ephesians: "Husbands, love your wives, as Christ loved the church and gave himself up for her, that he might sanctify her, having cleansed her by the washing of water with the word. . . ."[25]

Dr. Emoto's work reveals when the words *love* and *gratitude* are written on the inside of a glass filled with water, a picture shows that as the water reaches a crystalline state, it is exquisite, hexagonal, perfectly balanced, beautifully stable. When water in another glass is exposed to the word *fool*, it is nearly impossible to ascertain a crystal in what now looks like a mud puddle.[26] Emoto is clear: "We must pay respect to water, feel love and gratitude. . . . Then, water changes, you change, and I change. Because both you and I are water."[27] We learn from the Lord, himself: "Truly, truly, I say to you, unless one is born of water and the Spirit, he cannot enter the kingdom of God. That which is born of the flesh is flesh, and that which is born of the Spirit is spirit. Do not marvel that I said to you, 'You must be born anew.' "[28]

In the first chapter of Genesis, God's Spirit brooding over the waters creates all of life. John Indermark observes how, in Christianity and Judaism, water is a powerful symbol, bringing both good and damaging outcomes: in the Old Testament, Egypt and Mesopotamia emerged from the flood plains that were seen as a threat to human life, even personified as an enemy that God had to conquer; rampantly disrespectful human attitudes and behaviors preceded Noah's call to build the ark; in the Gospels, Matthew and Mark speak of Jesus walking on the water as an apparition or ghost; in Exodus, the waters parted and Israel escaped from slavery in Egypt; no matter their dissension, when Moses struck the rock with his staff, water rushed forth bringing life to the Israelites; and, when in exile, God brought streams of water flowing through the desert to sustain the people of Israel as they journeyed home.[29]

John baptizes Jesus; then, the Holy Spirit begins the deepest work of the Lord's ministry. The imagery of baptism in Christianity, so pure an act and expression of sacred waters cleansing and renewing us, often is given to mean the grace of God. The Lord God says to Ezekiel:

> I will sprinkle clean water upon you, and you shall
> be clean from all your uncleannesses, and from all

your idols I will cleanse you. A new heart I will give you, and a new spirit I will put within you; and I will take out of your flesh the heart of stone and give you a heart of flesh. And I will put my spirit within you, and cause you to walk in my statutes and be careful to observe my ordinances. You shall dwell in the land which I gave to your fathers; and you shall be my people, and I will be your God.[30]

Jesus is baptized and made known to us *in community*. God is well pleased with him, and we join Jesus in our baptism in which we are given our "name, grace, and calling."[31] In Christianity, the Sacrament of Holy Baptism is an outward and visible sign of an inward and spiritual truth. God says we are his, that our call, true identity, and eternal salvation as children of God are gifts of grace in love. In Genesis 9:12-13, God claims each one of us: ' "This is the sign of the covenant which I make between me and you and every living creature that is with you, for all future generations: I set my bow in the cloud, and it shall be a sign of the covenant between me and the earth." ' The Apostle Paul later writes of God's purpose in Christ: ". . . as a plan for the fulness of time, to unite all things in him, things in heaven and things on earth."[32] The Alpha and the Omega, all things are beloved of and belong to God.

Jesus speaks to the Samaritan woman at the well, ". . . but whoever drinks of the water that I shall give him will never thirst; the water that I shall give him will become in him a spring of water welling up to eternal life."[33] In his beautiful and scholarly book, We Walk the Path Together, Brian J. Pierce, OP, reminds us of the Judeo-Christian teachings that God creates us in God's image and that we are one in being with God.[34] The concept of one mind, let alone *mindfulness*, is ancient. Mindfulness may be a drop in the bucket. To be clear in mind and spirit, and to live lovingly each day is true sacredness. The work of the Holy Spirit is constant and to a depth most of us would think incomprehensible *once* and, with humility and humor we may be aware, *eternally* each moment. The more we are healed, and remain at-peace in the grace and power of the

Holy Spirit, the more humbling, joyous, and clear will be the Lord's work within and through us. We are united in Christ, with Christ, in, unto, and for the Lord God's eternal purpose in our lives, and to God's glory and honor and praise. Thanks be to God.

Writing of the 13th Century Dominican mystic, Meister Eckhart, Pierce reflects upon the paschal mystery of Christ's death and resurrection, and the awakening of the seed within us that "is watered by grace . . . and the seed of God grows to be God."[35] It is the Holy Spirit who gives, eternally anew, the power to rediscover our oneness with God, our true self, our reunion, in, of, and unto God.

The composition of water, the liquid component of all living things, changes when we cry. In his intriguing book, Crying, Tom Lutz writes of how, in over 3,000 years of representations in various cultures, we have understood and used tears.[36] Human beings can and will cry. Scientifically, we know tears of sadness have a different chemical composition than basal or continuous tears that lubricate our eyes when we are not crying. Researchers have identified the nerves that fire and the brain systems that are activated when we cry. Physiologists have studied the lachrymal glands that produce our tears, and researchers have attributed the production of tears to spiritual, physiological, psychological, and even medical reasons, and offering healing results and benefits. The chemical composition of lachrymal tears creates healing changes in the brain, resulting in total body healing for the grieving person.

The earliest record of crying denotes the "separation cry" as being the one between mother and child.[37] Lutz notes Darwin's observation that "weeping is one of the 'special expressions of man,' crying a human peculiarity."[38] Parents know that no matter what provokes their child's tears, loving action is the only appropriate response. We are encouraged to remember the second commandment: love your neighbor as yourself; we need to give ourselves, too, kindness and a heart that listens to the quiet voice within when we are crying.

How could we *begin* to understand another's tears? Do our tears represent both the desire for and the fear of intimacy, and with whom? Our loved one? The God of our understanding? Ourselves? Perhaps all three when we are focusing upon grieving loss. The GBU letters suggest a confluence or uniting of these levels of being known, fully and immediately to ourselves, and by God. This is our soul connecting with the totality of God, being holy, sacred, known. Our deepest love is with those with whom we are given to share our true selves. I call this "4:56 a.m.," for it was that hour, 4:56 in the morning, when I accepted the grace to share my most fearful self with a loved one. Why are we afraid? What is this *water-pouring-down* from our eyes telling us? Defining the word, "anthropomorphize," may help us to better understand our feelings of fear.

We seem to know, intrinsically, that everything comes from love or fear. To anthropomorphize God means to attribute human form, personality or traits to God; it means we make God into our image, rather than to acknowledge we are, our *be*ing is created in the image of God. Is God love? Is the God of your understanding infinitely forgiving, loving, kind, present, encouraging, and giving in wisdom and generosity, patient, peaceful? Are you open to this *constancy of love* and its teaching?

> It is God who justifies; who is to condemn? Is it
> Christ Jesus, who died, yes, who was raised from
> the dead, who is at the right hand of God, who
> indeed intercedes for us? Who shall separate us
> from the love of Christ? . . . For I am sure that
> neither death, nor life, nor angels, nor principalities,
> nor things present, nor things to come, nor powers,
> nor height, nor depth, nor anything else in all
> creation, will be able to separate us from the love
> of God in Christ Jesus our Lord.[39]

Or, if you do not know *this* love, is your understanding of God based on fear? Have you experienced authority figures throughout your life as hurtful, even the opposite of the aforementioned attributes? In First John (4:4, 7, 18), we are told: "Little children, you are of God, and have overcome them; for he who is in you is greater than he who is in the world. . . .

Beloved, let us love one another; for love is of God, and he who loves is born of God and knows God. . . . There is no fear in love, but perfect love casts out fear."

As deep healing progresses, one of many miracles is evident: we become aware of when we are crying for the other, for the person, animal, dream, the loss, itself, versus when we are crying for ourselves in relation to or, much less consciously, in relationship with that loss. The difference becomes profound, and is what I call "a marker" of our intrinsic, foundational growth, maturity, and healing; it offers a *glimmer of knowing* the Lord's love *with us* through our suffering of loss. Tom Lutz comments upon the repeated manner of depicting, over centuries of paintings, Christ's crucifixion and deposition (lowering the deceased body of Jesus from the cross): "Often a woman will look in anguish at the cross or at Christ's body, while others, weeping, look away. Crying allows us to turn away from the cause of our anguish and turn inward, away from the world and toward our own bodily sensations, our own feelings. Our feelings overwhelm the world, or at least our ability to process any new information from our world."[40] Quixotically, even as "a hart longs for flowing streams," and we thirst for God, seeking the face of God, still we know the pain of our tears having been our only sustenance; people may ask, "Where is your God?"[41]

Often, in grieving, we feel separate from others. We may want to remain distant, to protect ourselves from the realities of the loss. Neurological changes in the brain accompany every human feeling; correspondingly, physiological changes in the body accompany our tears. Tears may be seen as a *synecdoche,* a metaphor in which a part stands for a whole.[42] The feeling of life not being present to us, experiencing a surreal quality to just about everything we think or do during a time of grieving, is what I term being in *the Jell-O pool.*

The Jell-O Pool

Getting back in the river, used as a metaphor in bereavement, suggests a loss has the power, almost literally, to *yank us out of the water*, out of the ebb and flow of life. Nearly everyone who experiences the death of a loved one, or realizes their own life or the life of another has changed irrevocably (for example, from a stroke, Alzheimer's Disease, personal injury, or birth-related change in development or possibility), knows the feeling of what I call being in the swimming pool of Jell-O. In *the Jell-O pool*, we look up, see the world continuing, and ask, "How can that be?" The birds are singing, people go on with daily life. We feel slowed, invisible, somehow buoyed and carried along, yet, not present or actively participating. We feel unable to move forward in the manner and timeliness of our own desiring. We cannot abide feeling we are in *the Jell-O pool* for very long. We want to get out of the pool and the sooner the better. We may prefer to remain in *the Jell-O pool*. Why, at a less-conscious level, would we choose to be in *the Jell-O pool*?

After a death, *getting back in the river*, being present in life, requires that we *actually do something* about the loss. We may feel numb, be angry with God, feel upset with others or ourselves and especially with those who survived the loss (persons who are still in life as we knew it), even to the point of experiencing survivor's guilt, unsure of what to do next. We may pray and not see the way in which the Lord can help; we are called to be faithful. We are not embracing our grief because we do not recognize it. It is probable we are suppressing or repressing our feelings or remaining in denial about them.

Ungrieved loss can "sit" or remain a less-conscious barrier to life for 20 years, even double or triple that amount of time. If we have just emerged from *the Jell-O pool*, no matter how present we remain, we do not want to hear any reminders about the loss, beloved or not. After all, we are doing okay, right? Keeping busy . . . which helps us think about "it" less. Yes? At least for awhile; again, "awhile" can be hours, days or many years. Glib remarks often result in continued denial about the loss, itself, *or* its impact in the life of the grieving person.

Thoughtful comments from others may include: "You know your loved one is with God," or "They are better off, now, out of pain," or relieved of a serious struggle the person had experienced. Most of these well-meaning statements are spoken in kindness. All too frequently, the loss-survivor will dive right back in *the Jell-O pool,* instantly. Significant effort is required to heft ourselves out of *the Jell-O pool* or, gradually, to make our way to the shallow end with the intent of leaving *the Jell-O pool* behind and going on with life. Multiple levels of meaning are contained in our grieving of a loss that is important to us.

Sadly, we may be in *the Jell-O pool.* What are we to do? Life-changing, inner healing often occurs when we leave the shallow end of the emotional *pool* and risk moving to the murky depths of our emotions. The difference is one of quantum significance. Remaining in *the Jell-O pool,* being more than our normatively unconscious selves, yet, *seemingly* safe, comes at a great cost to us as the grieving person. We are not even close to the river at this point, let alone to *getting back in the river.* If we were in a pool filled with water, the outcome could be quite different. When we swim, paddle or float, the water, itself, and changes in the neurochemistry of our brain offer possibilities of deep healing, of beginning life anew; still, we may feel alone.

I have met with clients in psychotherapy who have remained in *the Jell-O pool* for 20 years, 33 years, 38 years, and 46 years, while totally blocking, repressing or denying the life impact of *the loss.* The effects are staggering: a beautiful woman who lost all of her teeth from grinding them, prior to asking for help 45 years later, long after the end of one family member's abuse of another which my client had not discussed until entering therapy over 10 years ago; individuals and families who remain in substance-abusing or otherwise-addicted lifestyles, losing everything and everyone, sometimes more than once, and themselves, daily; bright and creative men and women who continue to make less than wise choices, and, instead, for years, remain anxious, depressed or dysthymic (long-term, low-level depression). Until we acknowledge and own the loss, little will change except that we will experience an increase in the very

21

real possibility of gradual, personal death and/or the loss of healthy, interpersonal relationships.

Dying to Self

Grieving death is the most difficult thing we can do in life. *Healing* loss, and especially a loss significant to each of *us*, is one of the last things for which we would volunteer. Our life, the life of the person who is grieving, has changed forever. Jesus tells his disciples, ' "I have said this to you, that in me you may have peace. In the world you have tribulation; but be of good cheer, I have overcome the world." '[43] Cheer? Jesus is taking us deeper and says, 'give me your pain' that I may give you God. It would be rare for us, the one in bereavement, to surrender at this point. We begin to lose any coherent sense of who we are or were prior to the death or significant loss. In the 17th Century, William Law used the phrase, "dying to self."[44] Dying to self is spiritual growth; it is not our physical death.

While we die to self each day we live, one of our greatest struggles is to acknowledge we are grieving. A bereaved person *actually is suffering* the death of a loved one or other loss. Those who have not grieved may encourage us to "move on or get over it." Instead, we can choose to accept love's sacred presence, infinite hope and encouragement with us in every aspect of life's journey, and work *through* our grieving. Our inner work yields a rebirth, a uniting within us of the sacred in all of life. God loves and forgives us, giving us a humble understanding of the grace of life, already deep within our souls, and we begin to forgive others. The miracle of all that is holy and life-giving is that *new* life truly emerges, and can emerge in great strength, peace, and wholeness. Seeking the grace to forgive, to walk in unconditional, agape love is *of* God. Wow; sounds exhausting.

A clue: bereavement work is energizing, not enervating. The gradual healing of death brings newness of life, it does not further take life; this is precisely what we do not trust. First, and initially, we do not complete the grieving process because we are afraid we will lose the person, forever. Second, it *feels as if*, in grieving, we will lose even more life and we cannot face that.

"With God all things are possible;" in the early stages of our grieving, we are *not present*, and we have not begun to know the love Christ so freely and abundantly lavishes upon us.

The GBU letters help.

It takes most of us a long time as we work through grief to understand that dying to self and *mindfulness*, an ancient term, are the work of the psyche or soul, integral aspects of life. In Romans 12:2, Paul encourages us to renew our mind, and we think we created cognitive restructuring. We might be angry with God, the deceased, ourselves or someone else. It is, also, and more powerfully, that we *want to be with* the beloved person or pet, or not surrender our past or negative attachment. All types of *trauma* first create negative attachment. The latter, negative attachment, absolutely becomes a true barrier to healing, to forgiveness, and to genuine growth. Job epitomizes our feelings that in surrender we shall be nailed to the cross, annihilated, left to die. In truth, as Job lived, we are given the grace to *let go* and, gradually, to become who God creates us to be in Christ. It is up to God as to what returns to us in newness of life: a former relationship is made stronger and healthier; a person who has gone ahead to "larger life" is restored in our hearts and minds, the event/dream/other we thought we were to "be/do" was simply a part of the path to God's deeper purpose.[45]

When we experience significant loss, we feel deeply saddened and may think or feel we want to die, ourselves, when, in fact, the emotional struggle is about separation. Attachment and feelings of rejection, versus attachment and feelings of disappointment, stem from vastly different sources and lead to vastly different outcomes.[46] Person "A," who experiences loss from a deficit and who has had a paucity of practice in working through "someone leaving" (emotionally, verbally, physically in death, separation or abandonment, especially at an early age and without what I term *compensatory nurturance*), often becomes *stuck* at a less-mature stage of development. Unconsciously, person "A" will behave in a manner the libido (our primitive biological drive) will register as pleasing; such goal-directed behavior actually expresses the desire for love. Without age-appropriate, respectful, safe, trustworthy, compensatory nurturance, person "A" experiences loss as rejection of themselves. For example, person "A" could become narcissistic (and narcissism is rare, thank heavens), saying a sentence such as, "If you do not give me what I (person "A") want, then you do not love me." Person "B" who *experiences loss* from conflict, where nurturing love and limits were in place, usually will have had experience and practice in parental love and approvals being blocked until healthier behaviors gradually are learned. Person "B" develops deep loyalty to her/his parents or attachment figures. Person "B" experiences loss as disappointment, even very deep sadness and disappointment. Person "B" does not experience the self as being rejected. Person "B" is able to grieve. Feelings in this realm of grieving necessarily include anger, an emotion that covers hurt and fear. Chapter Four offers guidance in working through these sometimes frightening, definitely off-putting feelings of anger, hurt, and fear.

The difficulty for person "A" is the immature self has no place to go: they cannot reject themselves, no one else is there and no one else is trustworthy. Rather than experiencing disappointment, person "A" remains *stuck* in libidinal behaviors, anything that feels good to them or blocks feelings of rejection. While person "B" ultimately will move forward through the five Kübler-Ross stages of grieving, person "A" will attach to the person who died or other significant loss in an unhealthy manner. Person "A" will exhibit deficit-driven behaviors and will seek to become like the deceased to gain, finally, their acceptance, approval, and love. Person "A" does not know, has yet to learn, how to express less-developed, more-primitive feelings of loss; person "A" does not know how to express their basic human needs for love and affection.

If you are or anyone you know is even thinking of self-harm or expressing suicidal thoughts, please call 911 (if you are reading this book and can call for yourself); thereafter, immediately access the help of a medical and/or mental health professional. Most of us push away any in-depth discussion of death, especially our own, even when our most fervent hope is for a peaceful and loving transition to larger life. Five *stages* of grieving (denial, anger, bargaining, depression, and acceptance) will go around and around until deep healing of the loss is complete, known to us by our ability to embrace its gifts. During the five stages, two *levels* of loss are occurring.

The <u>first level of loss</u>: The first level of loss, albeit we may not want to admit or feel its impact--it seems so simple, is that *we will miss* the person or dream. Examples of the first level of loss include: the house that burned to the ground or a seeming-opportunity that disappeared or a car destroyed in an accident, and the last example only after we know all survived and, we pray, are healing; or an inability to play a favorite sport which meant exercise, exuberance, alone time in nature or a relaxed sharing of time with friends. There is a vacuum, an empty place within us in need of healing. Initially, when we acknowledge we miss the loss, we feel less stable, emotionally, because we have not worked through our grief.

The *first level of loss* stems from our ego which may be understood to be the self in contrast to the world, serving as our conscious mind mediating between ourselves and what we understand to be reality, and working through our perceptions of and adaptations to reality. If the loss is important to us (*our* perception and/or reality of what it represents), then the truth remains: *we will miss* the beloved loss even when it may have been detrimental to us or when it had seemed to be an opportunity. At this early stage, we cannot begin to process and grasp the implications of the death or loss in our lives. It would be too much to ask. Denial is helpful at this point and such a glimmer of truth makes clear the experience of most people: grieving a death, through *its most hurtful period of time* will take 12-to-18 months.

<u>Complicated bereavement</u>, grieving more than one loss simultaneously or in close proximity, or multigenerational grieving, often requires lengthy periods of time.

<u>We evolve</u>. We can be present each day and live well; when grieving, we may not be able to connect at all. We change daily at every level: cells change throughout our brain and body, and we evolve *even in our experience of the integration* of our new

25

physical, emotional, and spiritual self in the world. The more-integrated self becomes clearer. It is true: we can connect with one another in moments, seconds, and in*deed* reflect instantly the depth and wholeness of God's Spirit within us. Even the well self thinks grieving ought not to hurt as much as it does hurt most of us; again, if the loss mattered to us, we will grieve. It is vital that we allow ourselves and make a decision to grieve. If we cannot embrace our grieving, then it is helpful to acknowledge our feelings, name them, not ignore or deny them.

Grieving a significant death or loss may take a lifetime and we cannot hurry the process; yet, we can cooperate with it, invite gradual healing, and remain present each day so as not to undermine ourselves. An arduous task, perhaps, and clearly one we *know* resonates with the phrase, "it's an inside job." Each one of us will grieve in our own way. We can remain in denial or become depressed rather than acknowledge or accept the absence of the person/loss. In working with one woman whose husband had died unexpectedly, the family of the deceased man was less than welcoming of her, as his widow, because, in real terms and unbeknownst to her or to them, *her presence reminded the family of his absence*. When the widow realized the impact of her presence, her very existence and physical life, and the physical absence of her deceased husband, she was able to move forward, to begin healing and embrace his family in its grief, also. The family connected more deeply and moved forward in being open to healing the man's death, a profound response, itself.

We store all of our memories with either positive or negative emotions attached to them. The first level of loss takes quite a physical toll. Repressing a loss or its significance is enervating, is consuming our attention and, necessarily, is using real brain power, neurons, to process these undesired feelings. Hence, even more energy is consumed, *spent*, to the point at which we feel depleted, lethargic, even passively or actively suicidal, *rather than* being able, in these cases, to remain in such an exhaustive state of awareness of the loss.

The second stage of the grief process, *anger*, seems to be preferable to being exhausted or to numbing, feeling nothing, or to feeling the sadness and depression of the loss. We may remain *stuck*: some thing you can't keep (see p. 65).[47] At least in *anger*, stage two of the five, we feel energized, less depressed, we feel something. Or else, uh-oh, back in *the Jell-O pool* or, possibly, forward into stage three, *bargaining*, which is our attempt to change the reality of the loss by taking a particular action. Enshrinement refers to actions that are obsessive in building memorials to the deceased person, animal, or other loss. Examples of enshrinement include keeping the favorite room of a deceased person exactly as it was prior to the onset of a debilitating illness or as it was upon their death; keeping all or most of the possessions related to the deceased person, pet, even a dream or an event; and, taking on character traits, hobbies, and behaviors to excess, of a deceased person.

Our feelings of agonizing loss stem partially from knowing we cannot bargain the person, pet or situation back into physical life, or undo any other type of loss. While the five stages will cycle around many times and in various order throughout our grieving, it is stage three, bargaining, that is the first to end or drop out of the process. For children, two stages of grieving are predominant: 1) anger; and, 2) sadness or depression (see Chapter Three). While *depression*, stage four, remains widely underreported, we do not speak of this mood state as being one of choice. In their excellent book, <u>Shadow Syndromes</u>, Catherine Johnson, Ph.D., and John Ratey, M.D., affirm that even one instance of depression changes the brain forever.[48] Conversely, we are flooded with information offering a variety of ways to lift feelings of depression that also change the brain including exercise, sunlight, healthy hugs, prayer and meditation, and, when needed or warranted, psychotherapy and medication, and transcranial magnetic stimulation. We welcome stage five, *acceptance*; it, too, is cyclical, and comes and goes throughout the grieving process. The five stages do not remain in order and every person may not experience every stage; yet, the cycle is familiar to most of us in grieving significant loss.

Bereavement consumes large amounts of unconscious energy. Complicated bereavement, grieving more than one loss simultaneously, frequently involves an insidious track: the delay

27

and sublimation of our feelings about the losses. *We **will** cope at all costs*. It is all just too much to deal with, so we do not. We do not want to be presented with the overwhelming task of taking responsibility for, learning of or owning deeper feelings about the losses, or calling upon ourselves to recognize deeper conflict within us in relationship to significant loss, or healing more than one loss at a time. Instead and unconsciously, we use defense mechanisms in order to maintain our sense of sanity. People rarely want to remain depressed, although the possibility exists that secondary gain is at work.

Secondary gain (the unconscious benefit to be gained in holding on to the loss) is powerful, *completely* unconscious, and protects our hurt or fear; it protects us from deep, unhealed feelings that could erupt in anger. We do not want to die, to self or in any other way; survivor's guilt is a part of this cope-at-all-costs, desire for life. Once recognized at a more-conscious level, secondary gain is perceived by the grieving person to bring positive reinforcement. It becomes evident as to why, during bereavement, we would want to protect ourselves from hurt or fear. Again, we *will* cope at all costs in a healthy or in an unhealthy manner. It remains an observation in clinical practice: when we hold on to the source of our grief or the anger turned inward, we contribute to significant levels of illness, from depression and anxiety to soma (body), medical illness. Or, we can own our feelings and embrace help in working through them with a bereavement counselor, in psychotherapy, or with a pastor or spiritual director, appropriately using medications when warranted. Positive actions offer support as we move through the grief cycle and begin to create necessary new life directions. The GBU letters are a positive choice: the letters move us to the point at which we become *unstuck* and absolutely can reveal our secondary gain. Since we are the only reader of the first of the two GBU letters and it is our choice as to whether or not anyone reads the *second* letter, we have much to gain in the safe, open, and private expression of our feelings of deep hurt in the first letter, thus surrendering them to God.

Many variables affect *dying to self* in the grieving process:
+ Length of the relationship;

+ Nature of the relationship before the loss;
+ Type of relationship;
+ When the death/loss occurred;
+ Implications of the manner of death or loss: age, illness, suicide, homicide, other life variables;
+ Presence or absence of support: family and friends, professional and spiritual connectedness; and,
+ Presence or absence of relationship with God.

The <u>second level of loss</u>: The second level of loss emanates from the sacred self. We can continue to grieve, become *stuck* in grieving, and remain disconnected forever from the loving Spirit and spiritual gifts of the deceased person, animal, life event or even possession. We can "choose" not to trust ourselves or another or, unwittingly, to believe the sacredness of love cannot bring about our healing. Or, we can remain open, forever, to the gifts of God in the loss, and to where these gifts offer integration and healing to the deepest parts of the inner self. The quiet voice of the Holy Spirit becomes clearer within us. God's grace and higher purpose become unmistakable, known to us, and our acceptance is authentic and true: *<u>blessings in the loss hold real and true gifts for the soul</u>*. The grace-filled gifts in the loss *are* the Holy Spirit's formation of our more integrated, whole, healing, emerging, and evolving sacred self.

A kindness and the true wisdom in healthy self-forgiveness may be in not having to remember something or particular aspects of something related to the loss. A *dying to self* may be this subtle and gradual, or more obvious and hurtful. You could be the rare person who has worked forward through life, all is behind you and forgiven, all of the meanings of your life learnings have been understood and integrated, and you are wise and deeply healed. You are either nearing age-100, and/or you have accepted God's grace every minute of your life. Perhaps, in our time in history, this healthy outcome has begun to be realized to a greater degree and by a higher number of people, although some die at age-95 *without* this gift of life healing and integration.

What helps most and <u>creates connectedness</u> during the grieving process is our honest, caring, and attentive presence.

Listen to the person who is grieving, and offer any form of nurturance while encouraging the grieving person to do as much for themselves as is kindly and reasonably possible.

As *we* grieve, we are encouraged to:

+ Express our feelings, respectfully and honestly, about the loss and its meaning to us;

+ Build a healthy network of family and friends;

+ Begin a more-conscious process of creating balance in our life;

+ Create and share meaningful rituals;

+ Talk about the person, pet, dream, event or other loss; as needed, compartmentalize;

+ Establish ongoing follow-up with friends or family during the first year and beyond;

+ Foster patience: with ourselves, as the grieving person, and with others;

+ Gradually assume new ways of being, of living life, in the present;

+ Be thankful for our life and its opportunities for renewal; and,

+ Enlighten our sacred, spiritual being.

Over time, the real tragedy in a person's life, albeit an example to others of what *not* to do, is when the gifts of a grieving person are not developed, hence, not shared or given away. In Luke 17:20-21, the Lord is asked when the kingdom of God is coming; Jesus responds, "The kingdom of God is within you." Margaret Mead, well-known, 20th Century anthropologist who worked with people living in remote locations around the world, remarked, "We do not know of a culture without a word for Spirit."[49]

Since these truths bespeak the sacredness of each person, the Spirit of God within, why would anyone *not* want to heal that which keeps us separate from our soul, our inner peace, from *getting back in the river*, from honoring God, humbling ourselves, and living our lives in the power of the Holy Spirit within us to God's glory and honor and praise? The Holy Spirit guides us in seeking God, brings our next step, helps us to walk in the gift of faith in Christ, and develops loving relationship with Jesus and one another. The deepest answer to the former question (why would anyone, we, *not* want to heal that which keeps us separate from God, our soul, our inner peace, from getting back in the river?): fear, secondary gain, an incomplete understanding or the absence of any lived experience of grace, of love. We carry our learnings within us, hopefully accepting the grace to eternally and quietly share them with others; we have the ability to relearn and heal as deeply. It is truth and pure blessing that, "Nothing can separate us from the love of God."[50]

Beginning Life Anew

Chapter Two

If you want to get rid of something, you must first allow it to flourish.

Lao-Tzu

Beginning Life Anew

Chapter Two

Defining the Good, the Bad, and the Uglies

Good, Bad, and *Uglies,* what a strange concept. Twenty-one years ago, when my Mom died and my then-written letters evolved to become the GBU letters, the term had not been bandied about and most would have associated it with the Clint Eastwood movie of a nearly identical name.[1] Writing the GBU letters serves a very particular purpose: to help us heal the deepest wounds of *ungrieved* loss, known to us, perhaps, at some level of conscious awareness (friends and family may notice our bereavement symptoms), and to help us choose to accept sacred love, ever present in the loss.

Misinformation about bereavement is rampant and may be summarized in six "dictums," as noted by John W. James and Frank Cherry:

1) Bury your feelings;
2) Replace the loss;
3) Grieve alone;
4) Give "it" time;
5) Regret the past; and,
6) Do not trust.[2]

Strong statements about a process, grieving, most of us would rather avoid; rarely, are we successful in doing so. It is a truth: if a particular loss is important to our healthy growth and development, "it" will continue to come around and around, presenting itself for our inner work until we work through it, thereby beginning a foundational part of our core healing. Completing the GBU letters contributes to our deep healing of loss.

The GBU letters are comprised of *two* parts, two letters: the first letter, the part from which the *good, bad,* and *uglies* name is derived, is a letter written by the person who is grieving the loss *to someone or something else*, the focus/foci of the loss. The second letter is written only ***after*** *three whole days* have transpired from completion of (and safely burning) the first letter or anytime -- 72 hours or greater -- thereafter.[3]

In Matthew, we learn:

> Then some of the scribes and Pharisees said to him, "Teacher, we wish to see a sign from you." But he answered them, "An evil and adulterous generation seeks for a sign; but no sign shall be given to it except the sign of the prophet Jonah. For as Jonah was three days and three nights in the belly of the whale, so will the Son of man be three days and three nights in the heart of the earth. The men of Nineveh will arise at the judgment with this generation and condemn it; for they repented at the preaching of Jonah, and behold, something greater than Jonah is here."[4]

The first letter, once written and read, is to be placed in an envelope and burned, a safe fire, a safe manner of burning the letter, being of paramount concern (see Sample First GBU Letter, p. 95).

The second letter is written by the person who is grieving the loss *to themselves from* the person, pet, event or material loss addressed in the first GBU letter (see Sample Second Letter, p. 95). Chapter Two describes the specific processes of writing the GBU letters and offers examples of the profound healing realized in writing them.

What are the definitions of the terms *good*, *bad*, and *uglies*, in the context of the GBU letters? The *good*: anything we liked or loved about the loss. The *bad*: anything we did not like about the loss. The *uglies*: anything we hated, the worst-of-the-worst in thought and feeling we did not want to think or feel, AND the thoughts and feelings that surprise us or those we would not think possible coming from *us*: that is, anything ugly/hurtful to the loss or to ourselves in our relationship with the loss. It is helpful to ask the staple questions of journalistic writing, *who, what, when, where,* and *how,* to understand the purpose the two letters serve. Answering each of these inquiries about the GBU letters helps to explain what they mean and helps us to remain present during a process of grieving that, almost by definition, moves us to a less-conscious place within ourselves.

It is likely we are confused, numb. In the best-of-the-worst situations (a loved one who suffered with a long and/or painful illness, an injury or "life condition"), we may remain so busy in taking care of things that we delay our grieving for an extended period of time. We may be afraid, angry, in *the Jell-O pool* (p. 20), unwilling or unable to embrace our healing: who cares, why bother, leave it alone (we, ourselves, often are left to grieve alone); God? God let this happen, why would I want to pray or seek God at all? Leave me alone! After all, the person left, the dream is gone, right? We do not see the resurrection, as yet; it may feel to us as if it is Holy Week, and too much like *Good Friday*.

In Philippians, Paul writes:

> Finally, my brethren, rejoice in the Lord. . . . But whatever gain I had, I counted as loss for the sake of Christ. Indeed I count everything as loss because of the surpassing worth of knowing Christ Jesus my Lord. For his sake I have suffered the loss of all things, and count them as refuse, in order that I may gain Christ and be found in him, not having a righteousness of my own, based on law, but that which is through faith in Christ, the righteousness from God that depends on faith; that I may know him and the power of his resurrection, and may share his sufferings, becoming like him in his death, that if possible I may attain the resurrection from the dead. . . . but I press on to make it my own, because Christ Jesus has made me his own. Brethren, I do not consider that I have made it my own; but one thing I do, forgetting what lies behind and straining forward to what lies ahead, I press on toward the goal for the prize of the upward call of God in Christ Jesus. Let those of us who are mature be thus minded; and if in anything you are otherwise minded, God will reveal that also to

> you. Only let us hold true to what we have attained.
> Brethren, join in imitating me, and mark those who so
> live as you have an example in us.[5]

The GBU letters help us *to know* God's love, mercy, and
forgiveness. Still, we are grieving; when we become aware of
this truth, honestly and kindly within ourselves, we are firmly
on the path of beginning our healing. This book offers an
enriched understanding of *grieving*, and a tried-and-true, sacred
manner from which to heal loss. We are called to surrender our
selves, our loss, the *dying to self*, to God. Jesus, God incarnate,
in the power of the Holy Spirit's actions of love and mercy, is
calling us to walk in faith. In loving action, the Lord's presence
shows us *how* to be an umbrella of faith when faith is not or
seems less evident in another; even, to *be faithful with* one
another as God in Christ is *with* us.

> As for the man who is weak in faith, welcome him, but
> not for disputes over opinions. . . . Who are you to pass
> judgment on the servant of another? It is before his own
> master that he stands or falls. And he will be upheld, for
> the Master is able to make him stand. . . . None of us
> lives to himself, and none of us dies to himself. If we
> live, we live to the Lord, and if we die, we die to the
> Lord; so then, whether we live or whether we die, we are
> the Lord's. For to this end Christ died and lived again,
> that he might be Lord both of the dead and of the
> living.[6]

On the cross, Jesus, as the God-man who is more ego-
identifiable to us, is dying for our sins, to his full humanity in
this life with us; then, by the power of the Holy Spirit, Jesus is
raised up and is, as always, one with God. We do not
comprehend God's action in the resurrected Christ, the Person
of Jesus at every moment, even though as baptized Christians
we are called to discern and to be faithful, really to accept the
faithfulness of the Holy Spirit, the Christ of our being. At this
point, it may be quite arduous for us to walk in faith and to
surrender our doubt.

We question whether or not we will be with this beloved person ever again; we feel our loss in their death and not our oneness with God and with our loved one in the power of the Holy Spirit. If one way of knowing the Holy Spirit within is to discern God's righteousness, *faithfulness, the gift of love in the struggle*, then we are called to surrender the loss immediately, give it to the Lord, for God's purpose to be served. We know the gift of love *in the struggle* at any moment in time, as we walk in truth with the Lord and are united with the gifts in the loss. In a seminary class, it was said that the Holy Spirit not only is with us in the struggle, more truly is the struggle. These understandings are akin to the words, "and God" or "because God" or "with God."

Jesus speaks to the centurion and to us: ' "Go; be it done for you as you have believed." And the servant was healed at that very moment.'[7] The GBU letters offer a way, with openness and honesty, for us to express and surrender our fear that we may lose the loss or not survive its separation from us. God's love brings our healing.

Writing the First of Two GBU Letters

Who, What, When, Where, and How

Who writes a GBU letter? From children to the very elderly, anyone can compose these letters. The most salient criteria are that the person not have unhealed brain damage (organicity or brain injury) or, otherwise, be unable to remain present when experiencing thoughts and feelings that have been kept out of sustained awareness.

Too often in bereavement, we think we cannot move forward, genuinely heal, and feel better. Three fundamental precepts guide my clinical work as a spiritual person and healer: first, *the soul is one with all sacredness in life*, the One we call God, immanent and transcendent sacred presence and power, and God can do anything; second, the Latin phrase, primum non nocere, which means, *first do no harm*; and, third, *no safety, no growth*. In grace we learn the truth of these three precepts. God invites us: "I am the way, and the truth, and the life."[8] God's

39

eternal presence with us, and always as the supreme healer in and through our sadness, despair, and struggle, unites us with the sacred, eternal gifts in our loss. The three precepts, above, describe holy love, throughout life, AND our well direction in life, our way of being and becoming. God keeps teaching us that *nothing* can separate us from the love of Christ.

In the eighth chapter of Romans, Paul reveals:

> Likewise the Spirit helps us in our weakness; for we do not know how to pray as we ought, but the Spirit himself intercedes for us with sighs too deep for words. And he who searches the hearts of men knows what is the mind of the Spirit, because the Spirit intercedes for the saints according to the will of God. We know that in everything God works for good with those who love him, who are called according to his purpose. For those whom he foreknew he also predestined to be conformed to the image of his Son, in order that he might be the first-born among many brethren. And those whom he predestined he also called; and those whom he called he also justified; and those whom he justified he also glorified. What then shall we say to this? If God is for us, who is against us? He who did not spare his own Son but gave him up for us all, will he not also give us all things with him? . . . Is it Christ Jesus, who died, yes, who was raised from the dead, who is at the right hand of God, who indeed intercedes for us? Who shall separate us from the love of Christ?[9]

<u>To whom</u> is a GBU letter written? A GBU letter can be written to anyone, even to yourself. If you are writing to another person, the person (or animal, event) may be alive or deceased. The person may bring fond memories to your mind, or not. One person asked whether or not a GBU letter could be written to someone who is alive and thought to be the cause of the death of another person (or your dream, pet, event)? Yes, and any other set of circumstances.

Again, Paul teaches us:

You will say to me then, "Why does he still find fault? For who can resist his will?" But who are you, a man, to answer back to God? Will what is molded say to its molder, "Why have you made me thus?" Has the potter no right over the clay, to make out of the same lump one vessel for beauty and another for menial use? What if God, desiring to show his wrath and to make known his power, has endured with much patience the vessels of wrath made for destruction, in order to make known the riches of his glory for the vessels of mercy, which he has prepared beforehand for glory, even us whom he has called, not from the Jews only but also from the Gentiles? As, indeed, he says in Hosea:

"Those who were not my people

I will call 'my people,'

and her who was not beloved

I will call 'my beloved.' "

"And in the very place where it

was said to them, 'You are

not my people,'

they will be called 'sons of the living God.' "[10]

<u>What</u> is written in a GBU letter? The degree of complexity of thought each person writes in the GBU letters will vary, and if more than one "set" (two) of letters is written, each set may be quite different from its predecessor(s). In general, younger individuals will compose simpler letters. What is written will be influenced by: the age of the individual when the loss occurred, the degree and health of brain development, the present age of the person, the circumstances surrounding the time of grieving, the truth of nature (heredity), and the vital experience of nurture (environment, presence or predominant absence of loving relationship) when the loss occurred and, it is vital, now.

The content of a GBU letter the child or adolescent writes often will be focused, poignant, and quite clear in its expression of anger and sadness. Chapter Three, *GBUs for Children and Adolescents*, presents a cogent, loving, and supportive procedure to guide parents in helping young people in the process of writing the GBU letters. While it is true that each of us moves through the grief cycle in our own way, Dr. Elisabeth Kübler-Ross defined five, universal, adult stages in the grief process: denial, anger, bargaining, depression, and acceptance.[11] In her foundational work four decades ago with children who were dying from cancer, Kübler-Ross observed that as primary processors, children usually experience two of the five stages of grieving common to adults: feelings of anger, and feelings of sadness or experiencing the loss as depressing.

The most important part of the <u>what</u>, the content of the first GBU letter, is the third column, the *uglies*: **what is acknowledged in the *uglies* column yields the first gold of the GBU letters.** A client, working through the impact of simultaneous losses, all significant life events, insightfully said, "Nothing acknowledged can be healed."[12] (See Sample First GBU Letter, p. 95, for a brief, focused example of the first letter.) Remember, <u>no one else</u> reads the first of the two letters, only its composer. The *uglies* are the worst-of-the-worst in thoughts and feelings about the loss we can express; any use of language, grammar, spelling, abbreviations or punctuation will suffice. *Our full and uncensored expression in the uglies column is vital to the healing power of the GBU letters.* Writing *half-hearted*, yet, deep-seated hurts and hatreds (fears) will not bring about true healing for the author of the letter. As a matter of fact, any attempt to "be nice to" or to "take care of" the person to whom or other loss to which the letter is addressed, absolutely will circumvent the deep healing evinced in writing the GBU letters. We betray ourselves if we leave the first letter in view for anyone else to read, *accidently*. We would not leave the first letter open for another to read if we knew its contents, even remotely, might hurt them; the same thoughts and feelings may be toxic to our own growth and healing.

Thinking about hurtful dynamics tends to perpetuate them, not heal them; write them down in the *uglies* column. When we are the survivors following the death of a person who is close to us, we may express guilt concerning experiences during the relationship while being reticent to acknowledge the deeper feelings behind them. The seemingly protective thought is that the deceased person, even pet or life event, will *judge* us for an unexpressed feeling. Deep hurt about the relationship may be lurking in our mind, and we have not worked through our feelings. What is true, and actually becomes our gift after the painful experience of a loved one's death, is the known-to-us depth of eternal love and growth present in forgiveness. The GBU letters help us to give the struggle to God; our choice to surrender is the healing work of the Holy Spirit.

When are the GBU letters to be written? Anytime. Some of my clients compose GBU letters within days or weeks of a significant loss, while others have waited 30 or 40 years or longer. *Higher order timing* signifies sacred time or *kairos*, ultimately, the will and way of God. It is healthy to be kind to ourselves in acknowledging a variety of feelings, some of which may be a surprise. It is in knowing we can choose how to express our feelings that we create further steps of wellness as we move through our grieving process. Each of us has a soul. When we are open to and ready for the healing only sacred love can provide, we embrace the Spirit of God. Our loving thoughts and prayers for healing join the heart of the Lord, whether the need is for us or for others.

In the Book of James we read:

> Is any one among you suffering? Let him pray. . . . and the prayer of faith will save the sick man, and the Lord will raise him up; and if he has committed sins, he will be forgiven. Therefore confess your sins to one another, and pray for one another, that you may be healed. The prayer of a righteous man has great power in its effects.[13]

The experience of over 2,000 people who have written GBU letters is surprise, almost disbelief, and a profound depth of healing love and forgiveness once the letters are complete, such that the prior, hurtful meanings *attached to the loss* are changed forever. If secondary gain is present (unconscious gain from holding on to the loss; see Chapter Four), the writer may not allow himself to be healed in the love and power of the Holy Spirit. The process of deep healing of the mind, spirit, and emotions, changes the brain forever. Research from The Mayo Clinic (January, 2009), introduces the concept of an "epigenome" which means "above the genome," and is understood to be "all the weird and wonderful things" yet unexplained in genetics research.[14] The newly understood concept of the epigenome makes evident our nascent exploration of the connections and actions of mind/body/spirit, all given to us as human beings who are created in God's image; hence, the vital importance of embracing whose we are and what we are called to do.

The when, the timing of writing the GBU letters is vital to the letter writer's outcome. We cannot, nor would it be respectful to force the writing of the GBU letters. Likewise, we can delay writing the letters and turn away from the sacredness offered, our inner growth, as these eternal changes in the brain will become well aspects of our mind/body/spirit. When a person takes prescription medication for depression or anxiety, experiences wellness from brain injury or active-addiction behavior, and the person begins to feel better, the medication, especially in combination with talk therapy, is producing changes in the brain that create healthier thoughts in the mind and newer emotions to do the deeper work of healing the loss. In his wonderfully readable and medically informative book, Change Your Brain, Change Your Life, Daniel G. Amen, M.D., clearly explains how the deeper limbic system and other structures of the brain affect multiple aspects of who we are and how we behave.[15]

Where does one write the GBU letters? Adults, adolescents, and children are advised to write the two letters in a familiar, obviously safe, and comfortable place. This might be a room in your home or another location that is quiet, relaxed, and already familiar. Emotional stability also is vital. It is best for an adult to be alone when writing the GBU letters; children and adolescents need privacy, too, and the nearby presence of a trustworthy person, someone they love.

How, exactly, are the GBU letters written? Each of the two GBU letters is to be *written by hand*, **not** on the computer or dictated to tape, unless a hand-written letter truly is impossible. If a person *cannot* dictate to tape or write, then it is imperative to seek the assistance of a safe and trustworthy "other" who voluntarily will assent to complete confidentiality. A format that works to help begin writing the content of the first GBU letter is to take an 8 1/2-inch by 11-inch piece of unlined paper, turn it to the horizontal view and draw two lines dividing the paper into three columns. At the very top of the page, write Dear _____, entering the name of the person, pet, event or other-named loss. Below the salutation and at the top of the first/left column, write *good*, at the top of the middle column, write *bad*, and at the top of the third/right column, write *uglies*. Where culture and language would begin the writing from the right side of the page, reverse the stated order. The content of the *good* and *bad* columns is best written from the more absolute, black/white perspective; no description is necessary, just a simple naming or stating of the *good* or *bad* "facts" about the loss (see Sample First GBU Letter, p. 95).

How much time is required to write the GBU letters? You may choose to pray prior to beginning your letters; likewise, with a child or adolescent. Most adults who can be alone with uninterrupted time will complete the first of the two letters in as little as 20 minutes or up to one hour. A further understanding is imperative for both the adult writing his/her own GBU letters and the adult who is supervising the child or adolescent who is writing the letters: full assent to *no safety, no growth. No safety, no growth*, means that the total safety of the writer is sacrosanct and foundational to healing, each step of healing, and especially to core healing (every cell in the mourner's body is healing) of significant loss. Create a quiet, peaceful, and relaxing place for yourself or your child, with few or no interruptions, during which time you (or they) can pray, and think clearly, openly, honestly, and safely about the loss.

Before you begin to write the first GBU letter, you may choose to pray that God's purpose is served in your experience of writing the letter and in your healing. A friend in graduate school, a Sister, had completed in a cross stitch design, the saying, "Prayer changes things."[16] Yes. When you have completed the first GBU letter, it is best to reread it once; then, put the letter in an envelope and seal it. The first GBU letter is to *remain unread by **anyone else***. You, as the sole person, the soul who composed it, are to be the only reader of the first GBU letter. Once you have placed your first GBU letter in an envelope and sealed the envelope, "burn that sucker!" When learning of this step, most people laugh heartily and later feel a release of tension in burning the first GBU letter, happy to be rid of the letter, knowing it will not be around for anyone to find and read. The first GBU letter may be burned in a fireplace or wood stove, in a grill, or in a metal can in a large parking lot on a relatively windless day; that is, it is to be burned without the remote possibility of creating an unsafe fire.

Once you have destroyed the first GBU letter in a safe manner, wait three full days, 72 hours or longer, to write the second letter (see Chapter Five). The longer you wait to begin the second letter (perhaps, within a few weeks), the more you delay healing the loss and embracing its gifts.

Beginning Life Anew

Chapter Three

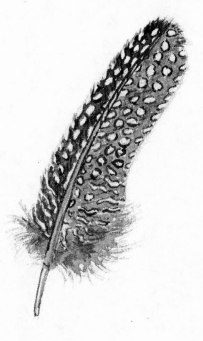

Treat people as if they were what they ought to be, and you will help them become what they are capable of being.

Johann Wolfgang von Goethe

Beginning Life Anew

Chapter Three

<u>GBUs for Children and Adolescents</u>

One marker of healthier families is the open expression of feelings and, in the area of bereavement, a willingness to talk about death as a part of life. Typically, such conversations focus on the death or loss of a pet or a move from one school or team to another (friends, activities), and the fact that nearly everyone will experience loss at some time (see Grieving Patterns by Age-Group, pp. 56-58). The adult who is *un*comfortable with death and loss is likely to convey inattentiveness to the grief response of a child or adolescent, and to ignore their expression of feelings. Most children do not go through all five Kübler-Ross stages of grieving death. Children usually experience feelings of anger and sadness or depression due to the fact that the loss represents significant change in their young lives, and they benefit when encouraged to express their feelings as a part of its acceptance. It is helpful to allow children to cry, to express their feelings of anger, and to respond in their own way, *while* reassuring them of three things: 1) you love them; 2) the loss is not their fault; and, 3) you are not leaving them.

When children and adolescents become angry, they need to express their feelings with someone who is safe for them and accessible to them. The emergence of an effective leader has been shown to encourage calmness, and to provide strength to people of *all* ages in the shock and panic phases of loss. To create stability, one helpful action is to *separate with safety*, a panicked child or adolescent (or lower-functioning adult), and offer simple commands to them: "Let's walk a little; you've had the breath knocked out of you, breathe as deeply as you can," (with the stomach relaxed as in yoga breathing; see p. 70).

Shock, panic, and even numbness (for example, not being able to feel, not being close to people, losing inner peace, clarity or strength, or momentarily not knowing how to respond) tend to precede the return of such feelings as denial (adolescents and adults), anger (anyone), and resentment (adolescents and adults). During times of undue quiet or turmoil, it is important for the child or adolescent to know you are aware of the loss, that Jesus/God also is aware and with them in their healing, and that their likely shifts in thoughts, feelings, and behaviors are normative expressions of grief.

It is helpful to engage children and adolescents in various activities during bereavement that offer different opportunities for expression of their most painful feelings in small doses. As the adult, your loving support teaches your children they are not alone, that loss takes time to heal and many different feelings are possible, and that they will move forward through their feelings of anger and sadness. As the loving adult, you can share, appropriately, with the child and adolescent that as the Lord goes before us, God has given you the blessed responsibility to love and be with them, to guide them through their periods of sadness, and to help them feel better.

Children

Children of all ages may express difficult feelings in many ways. Up until eleven or twelve years old, children struggling with death and loss may prefer or be encouraged to engage in one or more of the following activities:

+ Drawing themselves *prior to* when the loss occurred, and at-present;

+ Creating stories, puppets, games, paper/clay figures or other objects associated with the loss;

+ Drawing recent/recurring dreams, pictures of family, or a picture of an *uglies* feeling; and,

+ Drawing "house, tree, person" (themselves), and/or something scary or worrisome.

Overall, these activities need to be supervised with patience, and the child or adolescent encouraged to share her/his thoughts and feelings about them. It is important to *ask children to share* their expressions of grief (drawings, puppets, stories) as a means of conveying respect for their privacy. A variety of excellent resources exists on-line and in the library offering creative, responsible, and loving suggestions to help your child or adolescent work through their unique grief response. It is imperative to be aware of your own thoughts and feelings about death, and your child's particular loss in order to help them. If you cannot be helpful, then it is wise and loving to obtain help for them and for yourself.

When a child reaches the age of eleven years old, the child may choose to write a letter, including a GBU letter to the person, pet or other loss. Popular methods of *releasing these letters into life* include placing them in a balloon (which has negative environmental consequences); writing them on biodegradable paper and later making "boats" that can be released in a pond, river, stream or an ocean; and, burying the letter under a new tree or plant. With the nearby presence of an adult to monitor or supervise, the letters may be burned, safely.

Again, for children, it is vital that a parent or other trustworthy adult is nearby, providing safe, private, and uninterrupted time for the child or adolescent to write the letters. The supervising adult is NOT, absolutely not to read the child's letters. The caveat to the last guideline, that the child's GBU letters may not be read by the supervising adult, is that the supervising adult must be grounded in a realistic assessment and understanding of *primum non nocere*, first do no harm. Is the child physically well, for example, not home from school with the flu or a sprained ankle from soccer; and, psychologically well, that is, the child is *not* expressing thoughts of harming self or others, nor expressing a desire to join or be with the loss. If your child expresses <u>any</u> feelings of wanting to hurt themselves or a desire to harm someone else, or if you observe or are told about self/other hurtful behaviors, *please* call 911, or immediately take the child or adolescent to a hospital or to see their pediatrician, a primary care physician,

51

and/or a mental health professional for help (health department, wellness center, department of mental health or social services). If the child or adolescent gives any evidence, expression or behavior, of wanting to harm or to be *punished* (in contrast to healthy, *corrective* thoughts and actions), do **not** have the child or adolescent draw or write the GBU letters; please model calming behaviors and language, and seek outside assistance for the child and, again, for yourself.

No safety, no growth necessarily establishes an environment in which the child is emotionally stable, and capable of completing the letters with the *nearby*, yet, not hovering, presence of a responsible, loving, and respectful person who is available, if necessary, with nurturing supervision. The child may seek guidance, attachment or approval by raising questions as to how the GBU letter is to be written, how a word is to be spelled, or if such-and-such is okay to write, or, in the first letter, in which column does "this" feeling go? Answer each question as clearly and supportively as is possible. Any attempt by the adult to intervene, inappropriately, and casually to read over the child's shoulder, to keep a letter (especially, the first letter) for the child, and to be tempted to peruse and later to acquiesce to read this very private letter, will undermine the child's healing. The need to respect the privacy of the contents of the letter is just as important for the child and adolescent as it is for the adult. If you suspect, *at all*, that the child or adolescent is not stable, do **not** proceed; help them to be safe and to access professional help.

No safety, no growth describes even more than it stipulates, and it means that the total safety of the child or adolescent is sacrosanct and foundational to healing, every step of healing, and especially to healing significant loss. Once the child has written the first GBU letter, it is wise and loving to plan a gradual reentry for the child into the rest of his/her day with a brief inquiry, such as, "What questions or feelings do you have right now that you might like to talk about?" Most children will respond, "I'm okay, thanks; none, not now" or a version of this more positive response. The child may say, "I'm fine;" if so, genuinely work to engage the child in a dialogue about the *process of writing* the letter, *not* its contents. Examples might include statements or questions such as these: "Wow, that kind of a letter seems like it might be tough, hmm? No? That's good! How did it help you, Josh/Alicia?" Be prepared to name the loss if the child were to ask to whom you would write your GBU letter. Or, "That didn't take very long; how much of a surprise was it to be finished in __ minutes?" Or, "Gosh, the other step with this letter is to burn it, safely. Are you ready to do that or would you like to read it once, first? How shall **we** burn it?" If the child seems to be *stuck* (see p. 65), and is taking a long time to write the GBU letter, and, definitely, if the child has not joined you in 15 to 30 minutes, then, knock on the door and remain near the door while calling the child's name, and ask, "How are you doing?" Encourage the child to take a break if that would be helpful. If the child does not choose to return to complete an unfinished first or second letter, do not pursue that action. Instead, gently inquire at an appropriate time, "What are your thoughts or feelings about completing the letter?" If the child or adolescent asks you to read their GBU letter, you may help them by, 1) asking why this would be helpful to them, and 2) stating lovingly and clearly that you decline to do so, even if they choose to burn or shred what has been written thus far. With loving inquiry and support, you are grounding the child and reconnecting with them, making clear your respectful, safe, healthy, limit-setting presence with them. *Always* be loving and patient with your child/adolescent as you honor their grieving process.

Adolescents

During adolescence, many teens experience one-to-three deaths from among their peer group, family members, teachers, and parents or siblings of their friends. Frequently, the deaths are sudden and often violent: suicides, vehicle crashes when peers have abused alcohol or other substances, or overdoses. As if the losses, themselves, were not enough, their timing is superimposed upon multiple aspects of adolescent development, including changes in the brain that continue until the mid-twenties, with bodies that have begun to resemble those of adults in lives not able to assume adult responsibilities. When siblings lose a parent to death or to a divorce, or the grandparent who raised them develops an illness, the results may include diminished emotional support, shifts in role for every member of the family, exacerbated guilt during a time of normative adolescent separation, and role-shifts for the adolescent, absent the nurturing adult who would have provided unconditional love and support. These effects heighten the need for safety, acceptance, connection, and appropriate limit-setting at a time when teenagers too often experience rejection while seeking independence.

Symptoms indicative of an adolescent's need for help from a school counselor, mental health professional, mentor or other truly caring adult, include:

+ A decrease in academic performance;

+ Anhedonia or loss of pleasure in activities and interests the adolescent previously enjoyed;

+ Changes in mood and behavior, usually seen as depression, changes in sleep patterns, increased use of substances as mood altering "solutions," increases in arguing or emotional withdrawal, decreased interest in personal hygiene, clothing or overall appearance;

+ Shifts in peer group reflecting poorer self-concept; and,

+ Any lack of participation in former life interests.

Responses of loving adults can help the adolescent create a wide path toward emotional stabilization in what may be their first experience of death or significant loss. As will children and adults, teens *will* grieve, alone or with the support of nurturing others. Talk with adolescents, validate their feelings, and offer to help them join a grief support group. Be kind to them and compassionate, during what for most is a time of confusion and vulnerability. Often, adolescents experience a total shift in life meaning, along with the great likelihood that most, repeatedly, will push away offers to help them (see Grieving Patterns by

Age-Group, pp. 56-58). The adolescent may be your own or the child of another; in the latter case, when you hear or observe cause for any concern, speak with the other parent or supervising adult, approaching them with kindness and clarity. You may need to suggest, appropriately offer or obtain help for the adolescent or for the grieving family.

Hospice programs are available in many communities. Call to ask if your local hospital or hospice program offers a bereavement support program for children and adolescents. During such a program, a buddy or group leader can guide the adolescent group in gathering around a camp fire to share feelings about their lives since the loss occurred, to create a play or skit or game of charades, and to connect with their peers in open acknowledgment of their grief. Safe peer support in a bereavement group, with a buddy and a group leader serves as preparation for the adolescents who are ready to write their own GBU letters to the person(s) or other loss. Peer relationships, via electronic media or snail-mail, provide ongoing support for teens and when they compose their second letters.

Adolescents are fabulous and may be maligned during a normal process of growth and maturation. They will make it, most of us do; your loving supervision is vital. We simply want all people, and adolescence can be a difficult time, to know we love them, are always here for them, and they have not lost their minds during a time of utter confusion and unfathomable loss and life change.

The summary which follows, Grieving Patterns by Age-Group, outlines symptoms and patterns of grieving children, from one-to-two years of age, up through adolescence.

Beginning Life Anew

Grieving Patterns by Age-Group

Children and Adolescents

Children naturally express grief. Stages of life development in children and adolescents, and our inability as adults to recognize their symptoms and patterns of grieving inhibit our effectiveness in helping them to heal. The summary, below, identifies grief patterns by age-group.

1 to 2 YEARS of AGE

Three phases are common in response to loss and separation:

Protest: loud, angry, tearful behavior demanding and expecting reunion;

Despair: misery, depression, and a sense of abandoning hope;

Detachment: apathy, indifference to others.

Children of this age have no control over their grief reactions and express them overtly.

2 to 6 YEARS of AGE

Children may seem uncaring when confronted with death which does not mean the death had no impact; it reflects the emotional capacity of the child.

Children ask many questions about where the deceased person is and when they will return again.

Unexpectedly, children may exhibit aggressive behaviors.

Children act out emotions via tantrums or irritable and withdrawn behaviors.

Children may reenact the funeral or death via play in order to gain control of their feelings and make sense of the experience.

Children may make very blunt statements about the death at inappropriate times, shocking adults who are present.

6 to 9 YEARS of AGE

Children may use *denial* as a defense mechanism.

The tendency is that a child will not ask questions and will be able to maintain the denial by *not knowing*.

Many children behave as though nothing has happened; the outer life looks like nothing has happened, yet, the inner life suffers.

Because a child seems unaffected, support is not offered, resulting in repression of the mourning process.

Children of this age have strong feelings of loss and extreme difficulty showing it; boys, in particular, have difficulty, and frequently exhibit aggressive responses and play patterns rather than grief.

Guilt is a strong factor at these ages; children often revert to *magical thinking* and, in some way, feel they caused the death or loss.

Children from 6 to 9 years old need permission to grieve from caring adults in their lives.

9 to 12 YEARS of AGE

Children usually are shocked by the news of death.

Grieving patterns may look similar to those of adults.

Children will try to make sense of the death and try to come up with reasons to help themselves understand it.

Although there are great feelings of loss and grief, there is an equal need to present a strong, coping exterior; boys, in particular, strive to appear strong and in control.

It is easier to display anger and irritability than to open up; this may not be seen as a grief response, either by the child or by those with whom the child is involved.

There is a tendency to identify with the dead parent or sibling; the child may adopt habits, mannerisms or hobbies in an effort to keep the person "alive."

Children at this age must be encouraged, repeatedly, to talk about the loss and to express their deep inner feelings in order to allow mourning to result in a genuinely positive outcome.

12 YEARS of AGE through ADOLESCENCE

Common grief reactions include confusion, depression, guilt, shock, and anger.

These reactions are complicated by the changes all adolescents experience at puberty.

This age-group naturally exhibits great narcissism, ego-centrism, and self-preoccupation: traumatic events always are evaluated in terms of how the event affects them personally with little thought given to the impact on others.

During this period of increasing independence, the loss of a parent can be especially devastating: teens have to cope with the shock of realizing how much the parent was loved and needed at a time when moving away from them is a major focus.

Teens often dramatize their reactions, and use self-isolating behaviors: locking themselves in their rooms and not communicating, not eating for a day or two, skipping school or being hyperactive.

Temporary decreases in school performance are common.

Adolescents often test their "invulnerability" by challenging death through reckless behavior.[1]

Beginning Life Anew

Chapter Four

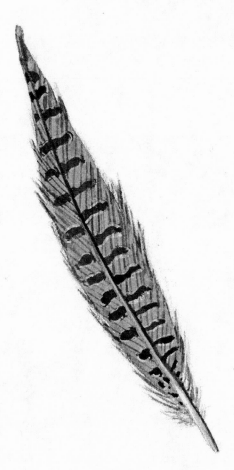

*If we really want to love, we must
learn how to forgive.*

Mother Teresa

Beginning Life Anew

Chapter Four

<u>Anger and Forgiveness in Healing Loss</u>

Understanding one very powerful emotion, anger, and one action even more powerful, forgiveness, helps us move toward the bank and begin *getting back in the river*. Scripture speaks of God as being slow to anger, as holding anger only for a moment, as abounding in steadfast love, and as being forgiving of iniquity and transgression, and calling us to be the same.[1] "The Lord is gracious and merciful, . . . good to all, and his compassion is over all that he has made."[2] We learn, ". . . for the anger of man does not work the righteousness of God. Therefore . . . receive with meekness the implanted word, which is able to save your souls."[3] In Hosea, God speaks of God's decision:

> I will not execute my fierce anger,
>
> I will not again destroy Ephraim;
>
> for I am God and not man,
>
> the Holy One in your midst,
>
> and I will not come to destroy.[4]

God instructs us, over and over, again, to put aside anger and to forgive one another as God in Christ forgives us:

> And do not grieve the Holy Spirit of God, in whom you were sealed for the day of redemption. Let all bitterness and wrath and anger and clamor and slander be put away from you, with all malice, and be kind to one another, tenderhearted, forgiving one another, as God in Christ forgave you. Therefore be imitators of God, as beloved

children. And walk in love, as Christ loved us and gave himself up for us, a fragrant offering and sacrifice to God.[5]

In his prayer to Abba, his Father, the Lord asks that our trespasses be forgiven, as we forgive those who trespass against us.[6] God forgives us. Upon the death of Jesus on the cross, arms outstretched and reaching to the whole world, Luke conveys an *understanding* of the Lord's mind, heart, and purpose in sanctifying grace, in these words: 'And Jesus said, "Father, forgive them; for they know not what they do." '[7]

How very true; we do not know, even minutely, what we do to aggrieve God, or we would not do it. Too often, as someone once said, we *all* learn the hard way. We are given our emotions and we have dozens of them; it is more, what we do with them, how we use them. *Our learning is made visible in how we act*: do we think, sending out healthier chemicals in that brain of ours, creating well emotions and then positive behaviors? Sometimes, it *feels* as if our feelings use us when, indeed, the instructive power in our emotions often emanates from a crucible-like experience. Long aspect of our journey though it may be, the teaching our emotions offer (and anger is one of the most potent) opens the path for depths of learning and incredible forgiveness.

Anger and forgiveness contain their own gifts: the first, anger, while a neutral emotion, may serve as a barrier, not only being the talisman of other feelings or actions; the second, forgiveness, is the very action of God, the very breath and ground of love, uniting us at any moment in beginning life anew. **Ultimately, anger protects and forgiveness unites**. The content of this chapter addresses the purpose these two powerful relationship dynamics serve in bereavement, and encourages us to work through our anger, to continue to forgive, and to embrace the gifts intrinsic to grieving our loss.

It is understandable that we question whether our normative guilt as we grieve a death, a loss, might keep God from forgiving us. We have been separated from the loss, desired or not. Either way, we are still here, in this part of life, with an opportunity to make amends, forgive, and heal; survivor's guilt is an emotion with many applications. We may feel *separateness* from God; what does this mean in the context of writing the GBU letters? When we lose or are separated from someone or something we love, we may be unhappy, sub-clinically or clinically depressed, or extremely sad, because it *is* depressing to experience a significant loss. We may feel guilt due to an unacknowledged wish for the actual outcome. We may feel we do not deserve God's love and forgiveness; yet, we know love and forgiveness are God's healing actions within each soul. We can choose not to condemn or judge or accuse another person, ourselves, or something represented in the loss and, instead, in forgiving each other create new relationship. We forget that nothing can separate us from the love of God. Sigmund Freud may or may not be at the top of your list of favorite people; nonetheless, his concept of separation anxiety hits the mark in bereavement work. We may feel anxious, a physiological response to fear that is based in the amygdala, deep in the limbic system in the brain. The phrase, "fight or flight," describes actual, neurochemical prompts-to-action emanating from ancient parts of the brain when the feeling of fear is triggered.

As we move from denial to anger, we have just begun to recognize our separation from the loss. We could experience anxiety, based on the fear we are just beginning to feel: we will not see the loss, again, in the same manner. We may prefer being angry to being afraid. Deeply seated in ancient parts of the brain with a vital role in survival, anger is and has the power to function as a very passionate emotion. At least in anger we know we feel something: we are not in denial, nor numbed in bargaining, nor feeling depressed or sad because we miss the loss, and we have not reached acceptance from which we would hope to begin again.

We would not survive without the physiologically protective function in our anger response *when necessary for life*. Anger is maladaptive as a means of loving communication; essentially, it is an attempt to connect, albeit an immature form

63

of intimacy. While it may seem quixotic and confusing, we do not argue with people for whom we have little or no regard. Perhaps, we argue with what the person represents to us: the seeming loss of self when we or our differences of opinion are not accepted or, worse, disregarded or disrespected; and, the loss of relationship when another person, pet, dream or opportunity is ripped away or disappears, or is lost to us in another manner.

While it may not feel like it in the moment, no one can take our dignity and self-respect from us unless we give it away, in anger or otherwise. Why would we do so? We are called to surrender ourselves to sacred healing; to explore the possibility of a holy purpose in the loss; and, to discover God's grace as blessed, sanctifying love in the gift of death in life. At this point, we are identifying more with the *surrender to*, than with the *embracing of* sacred healing. We do not know where the healing path will take us. Clearly, we might prefer another way of teaching, of being taught, rather than what, initially, we think of as *surrender*. God's sanctifying love may be unknown to us. Remember, we are working through grief, something we struggle to acknowledge, let alone "do well," an unrealistic pursuit.

We are progressing when we move from denial to anger. It matters that we remember: anger is one stage of the grieving process. We shall move through this stage unless we remain emotionally or biochemically numb which would block the feelings that are present to help us heal. The passion of anger, at all levels within us, tells us *we* are alive. While normal, we are still in a regressed stage and we are *stuck*. Scripture admonishes us to relinquish our anger and to be at-peace. In truth, we are grieving; we cannot be honest with ourselves and skip this stage. A further difficulty is that anger covers feelings of hurt and masks another universal, primary emotion, fear. When we feel angry, the brain also is triggering the feelings of hurt and fear; ancient parts of our brain respond, *immediately*. If we think of the strength of three emotions, two of which are primary, simultaneously being expressed in a bereavement response, anger, and its hard-wired (and unconscious) role in survival, then, the emotional power residing in anger becomes evident; so, too, the reason anger is the stage in which most people remain *stuck* in grieving loss.

Stuck: some thing you can't keep. With sincere thanks to a client from many years ago for permission to use the term in my writings, understanding the use of the word "stuck" as an acronym helps to explain why it may feel better to *not* complete the grieving process. What is it we cannot keep? The loss; even our denial about the fact that it is a loss, keeps us from *dying to self* (see p. 22), an intrinsic aspect of bereavement, of death, of life. What are we to do? At an unconscious, neurochemically based level, our brain is telling us that we are angry, feeling hurt and afraid. Further, the fear is telling us to fight or flee. All we want to do is to forget about "it" or to move through the grieving process and heal our loss. This is our hurting or fearful self remaining *stuck*: we cannot retain our former self, perhaps, less-mature self, not wanting to feel or be alone. Such holding on is about negative attachment: at its purest level, letting go represents instability (moments, hours, days, months, even years) and the fear that we will not be okay, ever again.

God calls us to let go of our anger (Col 3:8) and to grow; to *risk more* intimacy, trust, and vulnerability, thereby creating deeper connectedness with God and with one another in humble truth, genuine understanding, and, often, laughter and joy. We *can* grow through periods of instability or chaos. How?

Paul tells the Colossians:

> But now put them all away: anger, wrath, malice, slander, and foul talk from your mouth. Do not lie to one another, seeing that you have put off the old nature with its practices and have put on the new nature, which is being renewed in knowledge after the image of its creator. Here there cannot be Greek and Jew, circumcised and uncircumcised, barbarian, Scythian, slave, free man, but Christ is all, and in all. Put on then, as God's chosen ones, holy and beloved, compassion, kindness, lowliness, meekness, and patience, forbearing

one another and, if one has a complaint against another, forgiving each other; as the Lord has forgiven you, so you also must forgive. And above all these put on love, which binds everything together in perfect harmony. And let the peace of Christ rule in your hearts, to which indeed you were called in the one body. And be thankful. Let the word of Christ dwell in you richly, as you teach and admonish one another in all wisdom, and as you sing psalms and hymns and spiritual songs with thankfulness in your hearts to God. And whatever you do, in word or deed, do everything in the name of the Lord Jesus, giving thanks to God the Father through him. [8]

In choosing to accept unmerited grace to evolve, we *act*, surrender to God with us, the Holy Spirit within, our fears, knowing they are temporal, not eternal. We learn: as simple as it seems, the most difficult aspect of our growth is learning to forgive, self and others, and to accept forgiveness. In our walk with the Lord, the quintessential exemplar of true love, the eternal teaching and learning of forgiveness is constant, joyous, and humbling in a way that unites us with God and with each other. Acts of forgiveness bridge chasms within us, and years and places in life where only love is the way of God to one another.

Yet, yet, actually feeling better honestly seems impossible. How can this be when we *do understand* so very much about grieving our loss? Each, grieving and forgiving, is a process, not a light-switch, as my clients often hear me suggest. We would prefer to jump right over the depths of our loss; if we do so, it is to our own detriment for we will have its inherent learning and gifts to discover at a later time. It may be a small step; whatever inner work is offered in the moment, take courage and act in grace, embrace it. Paul says to the Philippians:

I thank my God in all my remembrance of you, always in every prayer of mine for you all making my prayer with joy, thankful for your partnership in the gospel from the first day until now. And I am sure that he who

began a good work in you will bring it to completion at
the day of Jesus Christ. It is right for me to feel thus
about you all, because I hold you in my heart, for you
are all partakers with me of grace, both in my
imprisonment and in the defense and confirmation of the
gospel.[9]

The question arises: can we *think through* the loss?
Thinking, rather than feeling at this point, seems preferable,
although, the two are linked inextricably and precede our
actions. We move back and forth in our growth, thinking
healthier thoughts and creating healthier emotions; occasionally,
we take two steps forward and one step back. When we are
grieving, the cognitive process feels as if it is being derailed,
that *we are only* our emotions, and we are overwhelmed by their
persistent and chaotic presence.

Can we think through our loss, especially when the
emotions this bereavement business is bringing forward are
beginning to feel pretty ugly; ah, of course. In its exploration of
anger, this chapter was the most difficult to write. We do not
like to feel angry; nonetheless, the emotion exists to tell us
something. Anger *is* the second stage of the grieving process; it
is even stronger than denial, the first stage. Further, Paul tells
us, "Do not be conformed to this world but be transformed by
the renewal of your mind, that you may prove what is the will
of God, what is good and acceptable and perfect."[10]

As many of us know, even gingerly signing up for the
grieving process feels daunting. Again, Jesus embraces us
where we are: ' "I have said this to you, that in me you may
have peace. In the world you have tribulation; but be of good
cheer, I have overcome the world." '[11] Clients hear me say,
"Stay in a well direction, strength is within; keep the ground
you have gained in your walk with the Lord, be at-peace. While
growth is difficult at times, have faith, the Lord goes before us.
We are not asked to leave reason at the door of our inner work."

To recap, anger is potent for several reasons: first, it is
triggered, literally, in the deepest and oldest parts of the brain,
the amygdala and the hippocampus; second, it covers two other

feelings, hurt and fear, the latter (as is anger) being one of four primary and universal feelings; and, third, while neutral until the hippocampus confirms fight or flight, <u>the overall effect of anger is as a distancing emotion</u>. The problem: anger distances us from others, quite well; it distances us from ourselves, also. Anger works and works powerfully.

Picture yourself in the diagram, below, with the potential for a "fight" response to the right and a "flight" action to the left. Once the amygdala has been triggered, how can we intervene for ourselves and *think through* our response to an automatically triggered and neutral emotion that is necessary in its overt ability to protect us? See yourself in this picture and read the example question, which follows.

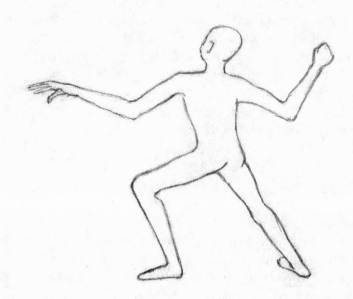

FLIGHT   FIGHT

68

Keeping the figure, above, in your mind, see yourself walking toward a concert pavilion or stadium with a member of your family or someone else you care about and love. All of a sudden, as you move together across a wide thoroughfare, a large, rapidly moving bus careens out of control and is headed speedily toward your family member. What do you do? Fight, meaning move forward and push the family member who is ahead of you out of the way, risking that you will knock them down, or flee, grabbing them forcefully enough to pull them backwards? Standing still is not an option. The neural circuitry in the amygdala is processing data about the oncoming danger in nanoseconds, even though the cerebral cortex has (yet) to be apprised of it. The instant signal from the amygdala literally keeps us alive as we move in a breath, a split-second. Again, what action do you choose?

As Joseph LeDoux observes in The Emotional Brain, the hippocampus and cerebral cortex can override the instantaneous distress signal with a "relax and recover" message telling our physical body the emergency does not exist; we relax and return to a more restful state -- most of us.[12] Today, we know the amygdala distress button is pushed easily, and often remains activated when someone has experienced ongoing emotional or physical neglect, persistent trauma or other forms of hurtful attachment. Anxiety, post traumatic stress response, even depression as a reaction to anxiety the person cannot seem to reduce, repeatedly will trigger the amygdala. With chronic stress over time, the hippocampus will atrophy and be less sensitive to the amygdala's signal to fight or flee.

It is widely known that our neural pathways contain the ability to grow anew in the adult brain, an opportunity called synaptic plasticity. Mental health clinicians encourage clients to develop healthy responses to stress or trauma that support actual healing in the brain (see pp. 81-83, the "Y-Solution"). Davidson and Fox, advocate that we develop methods of soothing ourselves, pointing to the practice of *mindfulness meditation* as a way to strengthen the left prefrontal cortex which inhibits signals from the amygdala.[13] We may begin to understand to only a minimal degree of what it is that St. Paul speaks: God works in us in the renewing of our minds; and, God "*has put eternity into man's mind*" (Eccles 3:11). Incomprehensible to us though it is, we are given, ' "For who has known the mind of the Lord so as to instruct him?" But we have the mind of Christ' (1 Cor 2:16). We are told (1 Chron 16:11): "Seek the Lord and his strength, seek his presence continually!" In Matthew, we find encouragement from Jesus, offered as a directive, with assurance:

> "Ask, and it will be given you; seek, and you will find; knock, and it will be opened to you. For every one who asks receives, and he who seeks finds, and to him who knocks it will be opened."[14]

The Lord knows our humanness, our mind, body, Spirit connections. To seek the mind of Christ, to surrender our fear and anger, we need to be peaceful or else our circuitry will not be clear. To breathe, to be present *inspiritus*, opens our brain and mind to the depths of the Holy Spirit within us. A very simple and effective technique I teach my clients allows the brain to return to rest *while* its synaptic plasticity provides healing, and it takes only a few steps and a matter of seconds. We may choose to practice this and be at-peace:

> 1) Breathe: *breathe*, pushing your stomach <u>out</u> <u>as</u> you breathe in <u>and</u> breathe out (ancient yoga breathing), being focused and intentional in keeping your tummy relaxed. This is a form of biofeedback: the rapid processor, our brain, instantly gets the message that blood is flowing evenly throughout our body and brain; hence, the brain is not being given the signal to fight or flee.

> 2) Ask yourself <u>one</u> question: *Why am I feeling hurt or afraid?* In concert with our calm breathing, the signal to our brain <u>is</u> that it is okay to continue in that peaceful mode, that we *are* addressing what is occurring, now, in front of us or in our mind that, formerly, could have triggered an acute anxiety reaction. The easier part of

the question is, *why am I feeling hurt?* Here, we can use our conscious mind: in the preceding example, we do not want to push or grab our family member (as we see the careening bus approach), and the thought of doing so is hurtful to us, a real feeling.

The tougher part of the question is, *why am I feeling afraid?* Hmm; we may begin with more-conscious thoughts and move to those at a much less-conscious level. I may not be successful in pushing the person in the right direction or far enough out of the way, or not in front of another vehicle I may not see at the time; thus, the other person might be injured anyway or in a worse manner, or those outcomes could happen to me or to another who is not in my field of vision. Wow. What *else* could be going on? In the given example, the person in direct danger is a family member or another loved one. If, in our split-second, brain-response-system, our action misfires or fails, what emotions would we be facing, then? Eventually, with loving attachment, we could heal our loss. During the interim, we would begin to deal with the ramifications of the loss event.

What if we cannot say we are angry? What if, instead, the action to help is blocked and blocked to the point where the opportunity to help has passed? Another emotion, *resentment*, could be the culprit. How can we understand resentment in the process of grieving loss? My definition of resentment is, *re-experienced, but unexpressed anger*; and, as we have learned, anger covers hurt and fear. The feeling of resentment may seem to be less hurtful to healthy relationships than the emotion of anger because it appears to be more subtle, openly acceptable, and may feel more tolerable. It is not, it is more lethal. Simply, when we feel resentful, we are *stuck* and we do not know it. What comes to mind is a memory of thinking, "It's their way or the highway," and realizing, finally, how often the thought had emerged: beneath the expression and the corollary emotion of resentment was anger.

What is going on? When one person presupposes to determine *choice* for others, interpersonal limits are placed on mutual respect and valuing, thereby limiting opportunities for individual expression and continued development. In any group dynamic, creative thoughts and actions also would be limited. Instead, embracing thoughts and behaviors that foster trust, honesty, respect, and clarity in relationships promotes a higher probability of better solutions among group members.

Let us visit a second, also real, example. The mom of several children brought the oldest, an adolescent male, to my office after the young man, uncharacteristically, had begun to kick holes in the wall and to be physically unkind to his younger siblings. Dad had left for the war in Iraq. Mom was at her wit's end: deep concern for their very loving family, with at least six months until, hopefully, her husband would return home. Many considerations seem obvious. In the first session, son and mom explained their reasons and goals for therapy, and discussed their family history; we decided to work together. In describing his behaviors, the teenage son was unable to articulate why he had become so angry, not to the point of denying his hurtful behaviors, yet, obviously unaware of deeper feelings behind his anger or resentment toward his dad who had left for Iraq when my client was fifteen years old. At the end of the first session, I asked the young man to think about the question, "Why am I feeling hurt or afraid?" and to pay attention if something were to come to mind or might come forth in his dreams.

In the second session, by himself, the adolescent was able to answer why he felt hurt. At the age of 15, he wanted to share more adult activities with his dad: sports, early driving experiences, not only being with his younger siblings, but with his dad, talking about guy *stuff*. Relationship with mom seemed positive and healthy. My client felt hurt that he would miss many opportunities with his dad, now that he was old enough to experience them. During the intervening week, the young man and his dad had made arrangements to connect via e-mail at least twice each week which greatly pleased my client. He said he had stopped kicking the walls. He felt, "honestly," that he was still being "too quick to get into arguments" with his siblings who were "usually okay, they're just kids." I encouraged this young man to think about the second half of my question: why was he afraid?

During the third session one week later, the update was quite positive: connecting with his friends at school, being proactive, and "better and more helpful" with his siblings and his mom (one of his goals); overall, reporting greater wellbeing. True progress. I asked the young man, "How did you answer the second half of the question?" My client was quiet and stared out the window. I waited. "He [dad] did not ask me how I felt about it" (the assignment to Iraq). Seconds later, a tear rolled down his left cheek, his eyes sad. Still, I waited. "He might not come back, you know, come home," said the mindful, struggling-to-do-his-work, young man. In a minute or two, he began to talk about his feelings of possible loss, his increased responsibilities at home, that he truly missed his dad, and his feelings of guilt when he did not want to share a family job because it "should be" his dad's role. His resentment, re-experienced but unexpressed anger, anger covering hurt: he ought not to have *this* task, too (any job his dad used to do). His fear: if he did not complete a given task and others to follow, how could he live with himself if his father were not to return home from Iraq? I encouraged my client to write the first GBU letter to his dad (again, not to be mailed, rather to be destroyed), with the second letter to follow, and encouraged my adolescent client to so-advise his mom. He wrote the first letter, safely burned it, and stopped his aggressive outbursts and behaviors. We met, again, with his mom. The young man wanted to receive the second letter from his father, directly. I learned much later that his dad had arrived home safely from Iraq.

Neither the first example of the family member at the pavilion event, nor the second with the dad being overseas, includes grieving the physical death of someone in close relationship. One such story is of a woman in her forties who had birthed two children, had had several internal organs removed, was divorced, and increasingly had withdrawn from her husband of twelve years while becoming dependent on antidepressant and anti-anxiety medications. She revealed that her mother had died when she was nine years old, and her hurtful, soma (body) responses had become worse and worse. However, the woman persisted in choosing to be well and her husband supported her goal. I diagnosed my client with Dysthymic Disorder (long-term, low level depression), and referred her to a psychiatrist who prescribed medication targeting her symptoms. Also, I suggested morning prayer, routine, mild exercise, and light therapy as needed. My client began to improve. Within two months, I suggested she write a GBU letter to her deceased mom which my client elected to do. The experience of completing both letters was described as "very healing and freeing . . . after all this time. I never thought that would happen." During therapy, this increasingly well woman related dreams of moving through deep levels of psychological, spiritual, physical, and emotional integration, indicative of more mature aspects of development. My client experienced core healing.

How is it we can begin to feel better when such losses occur? At first, we think the cost is too high or we have to get in touch with such seemingly destructive feelings. Or, worse, commit a terrible wrong in writing the *uglies*, putting them down on paper, the worst, hurt-filled thoughts and feelings we have toward a person. We question how anyone could dislike, even *hate* (fear) another person or an experience of loss so much as to carry around such ugly feelings?

We can choose to deny our strong, hurtful emotions toward another person whose loss we experience with varying types of pain; we will become *stuck* in anger or resentment. At least it feels as if we are still connected to the loss when we experience such passionate emotions. We do not have to peel away the protective layers to reach deeper feelings. After all, it was only Granny, Uncle Ted or Cousin Mary who loved us so much and may have been an integral part of our family as we were growing up. Yet, what about the fact that Grandma would not let us see mom or dad, even if Grandma were right to do so because of extenuating circumstances? Are we not more mature than that? Grandma or Uncle Ted may be 95 years old, now; how could we "say something to them" at this point in time?

We can choose to say nothing and write our GBU letters. What steps can we take to acknowledge our anger, hurt, and fear? Do we have preliminary steps to take? Breathing, praying, meditating, quietly reflecting, and learning to breathe through feelings of fear and anxiety are the first steps. We can revisit the decision to heal our loss as we keep breathing. Recognition of the effects or consequences of a loss may take months, years, even decades. If we have not moved forward in healing our loss and in understanding or glimpsing the gifts it offers, then we can be helped *significantly* by writing the GBU letters. Remember, the first GBU letter, addressed to the loss, is the letter that we, as its composer, *absolutely show to no one*; the first GBU letter is *destroyed*. The second letter is the one we can choose to share at some point, or not.

What if we do not want to forgive a person who died and whose death deeply hurt us, or a person who is alive and has become the less-conscious and enervating focus of our lives? Remember, our *un*conscious *always* is at-work; the distinction is vital. Michael Casey, Monk of Tarrawarra, "links the unconscious to Bernard's [of Clairvaux (1090-1153)] concept of 'the human heart', where God dwells and acts."[15] Maybe, we do not want to forgive. We can seek God's grace to help us; then, the choice to forgive is ours, and ours, alone. What will we feel when we let go of that passionate emotion of anger? Hopefully, we are at-peace, healthier, because we are *able to choose more consciously* to be present in the mind of Christ, in the power and fellowship of the Holy Spirit, and to accept the grace to choose self-care and loving, trustworthy relationships. Gradually and increasingly, we become conscious, bringing forth Casey's and Bernard's concept of the *unconscious* in choosing where, how, and with whom to share our lives.

Forgiveness

"Forgiefan" is the root of the word *forgiveness* and its meaning is "to abstain from giving." William and Rebecca Kirk understand "forgiefan" from the additive perspective, rather than from one of withholding, vis-à-vis "the importance and discipline needed to be a receiver of forgiveness."[16] Sacred to the core, when we abstain from forgiving another, forgiveness of ourselves is blocked as is acceptance of forgiveness from another. To accept forgiveness from someone, to be the receiver, is deeply and joyously humbling which can be experienced from the giving dimension, also. The act of forgiving signifies that we are grounded in our chosen vulnerability with another person because we are seeking loving connection and what the Kirks term "full relationship" with them. Much has been written about forgiveness and whether or not we need to forgive, the wisdom of forgiving another or ourselves, and our willingness to accept forgiveness from someone else.

Many of us have heard the phrase, "You can forgive, but you can't forget." Can we truly forgive and honestly forget? Yes. It is *a process of be*ing patience, *be*ing compassion, and *be*ing understanding. God calls us to forgive others as God forgives us. We are empowered by the Holy Spirit to be this love with one another. Forgiveness is a process: it requires our surrender to and joining with a higher love; it requires a choice, the act of choosing to forgive; and, it becomes a decision point, making the decision to change ourselves. The act of forgiving is *be*ing love, the *most* pure and kind reflection of God's holy presence within us (immanent) and with others (transcendent).

From forgiveness emanates core healing of every loss; it is how we grow in grace. With all of our human foibles, it is only in God's love within our souls that we, acting in grace, forgive, creating true peace and joy. The Holy Spirit indwells us, God is with us and, in grace-filled moments, we are aware of our loving and humbling oneness with the Lord. Forgiveness is the heart of love which is of God and is God in the Trinity, and in God's relationship with us. Again, God lives in community and calls us to do the same, to be unconditional love with one another, in, of, and unto Christ, in the power of the Holy Spirit.

What is to be gained when we move forward in our openness to forgive one another? We are in full relationship with God when we forgive. Forgiveness frees us from past frustration, hurt and fear, and from unhappy prior experiences and memories. Forgiveness reduces overall anger because, in the present power of the Holy Spirit, we have owned our feelings and claimed our internal sacred directedness, thereby rendering other sources of provocation powerless. We have increased our energy because we have released the heart to respond lovingly, consciously, to feelings of hurt and fear.

In <u>Man's Search for Meaning</u>, Viktor Frankl wrote of surviving torture in Nazi war camps, the diminution of culture, and the loss of his family and an untold number of friends. With extraordinary pathos, pain, and heart, Frankl said, "The one thing you can't take away from me is the way I choose to respond to what you do to me. The last of one's freedoms is to choose one's attitude in any given circumstance."[17] The knowledge that we have a choice in how to respond is one of the most consciously healing places of growth in human relationships and within ourselves. Choice focuses our attention on how we can be present with one another, makes us aware of our ability to create genuine connectedness in relationships, and brings self-acceptance, all of which increase our acceptance of others, creating the freedom to grow and develop as whole persons.

The actual process of *hand*writing the GBU letters changes the brain; true, neurochemical healing is taking place as we are anchored in life-giving forgiveness. As mentioned earlier, and it is the Lord's faithfulness eternally bringing this understanding to me, <u>when people do not complete the process of grieving the loss of a loved one, it is because they are afraid they will lose the person, forever</u>. Have you ever heard someone say, "I can no longer remember what s/he looked like." Perhaps, you have made that comment? Or, "I cannot even remember what s/he sounded like and I used to love to hear that voice. Ah, I cannot stand it! I do not want to feel like this one more day." Or, "I do not want to see that face, ever, again . . . hear that voice anymore. It is a good thing . . . good riddance!" Forgiveness is knocking on the heart.

What does forgiveness require of us? It requires that we *think* and think about why it matters that we forgive: that we are blessed to be able to forgive and to be given the grace to forgive; that we grasp this gift of God with us and in another which creates a deep sense of freedom and inner peace; that we choose, ultimately, to surrender to God who is love, who *lives in community* and calls us to do the same with compassion throughout our lives, no matter how we stumble along the way; and, that we are thankful, always, to God. Forgiveness creates love; and, love is the grace to forgive; it is *getting back in the river*, it is new life, at any moment.

How important is *understanding* in the process of forgiveness and what makes it possible? We seek and are given the grace: "both-and." Our *genuine desire to understand another person and to be understood* is vital to being able to risk the intimacy of mutual understanding because to create intimacy, in its depth of being known, is a choice we can make freely, responsibly, and appropriately; too, this choice comes only from the heart. When we choose to be open and vulnerable with one another, we create opportunities for greater depths of being known, of healthy love, in all of our relationships. Patience and kindness make forgiveness possible. It is not as much our willingness to permit another person to reveal themselves to us, as it is our gift and privilege *with* one another to be who we are created to be; ah, clearly, an eternal unfolding and discovery in our hearts. God is revealing God's love to us and with us in community. In abiding with one another, in near-incandescence, we can reflect God's love, "agapao" in ancient Greek, loving the way God loves.[18] It is impossible for us to love as the Lord loves us unless the Holy Spirit is present: Emmanuel, God with us.

Paul encourages us to renew our mind, to *think* differently, and, especially, to be open to God. Repeatedly, we learn: a) the mind is the supreme function of the brain; b) we are to renew our mind in as much health as is possible; and, c) our brain is the alpha and omega of our cognitions, emotions, and behaviors. In a theology class some time ago, it was said that the Holy Spirit is not *in* the struggle; rather, the Holy Spirit *is* the struggle. My more recent understanding of this offering is that when we *surrender to*, invite, and embrace the still, quiet voice within us, our mind is completely at-peace and we are not at all giving up, perhaps, giving over; we are one with God and God's will for us. The sacred forgives us and calls us to forgive others. Most of us would hope to live in the constancy of *this struggle* throughout our lives, abundant and eternal blessings of God. God calls us to forgive one another and ourselves. We can choose to forgive: we can choose to trust God's immanent and transcendent grace and power to help us to forgive. All is by grace.

Rethink Grieving

As persons, "we all carry grieving."[19] To be *beholden* to another means we carry real or a sense of indebtedness. Further, when we are open to teaching and learning together, we move to the depths of compassion: from the Latin, com- + pati, to bear, to suffer, be patient, sympathetic *consciousness* (italics, mine) of others' distress along with a desire to do what we can to alleviate it.[20] As we mature, we hope to evolve from being in relationships based upon dependence on another as infants and children, to those of gradual independence from others in adolescence, to interdependence with others as adults. Interdependent relationships call us to strive to share equally the overall responsibility for thoughtful and loving actions that nurture one another, in kindness, with full forgiveness, and personal accountability. . . along with our daily chores. If attachment has been disturbed such that needs were not met in a safe, primarily loving, respectful, and trust-building manner, then reaching interdependence becomes more difficult.

The grieving person who lives with unmet attachment needs and is attempting to let go, rethink, and trust inner promptings of sacred love will block the struggle rather than grow through the deep pain of loss. Accepting the grace to release indebtedness and to choose loving connectedness in full relationship with others enriches our souls, and we are more fulfilled and complete at that point on our journey and forever.

In the mental health field today, we have knowledge about the brain that was unknown fifty years ago. Greater specificity is available in our observations of the brain and its functions, via a variety of diagnostic brain scans (for example, MRI, CT, and SPECT), and from the effects of life-enhancing pharmacologic interventions, such as antidepressant, anti-anxiety, mood stabilizer, and anti-psychotic medications. With or without the effects of newer medical applications, in our bereavement work it is insightful to remember one of the oldest definitions of depression: *anger turned inward*. We forget that the word *psyche*, in Greek, means *soul*; why are we surprised? Thoughts are not cotton candy in the brain, but actual, neurologic activity with direction and necessary outcomes. In bereavement, the process of expressing anger, our feelings of hurt and fear, requires *real* energy, not only what we speak of as *psychic* (real) energy. Below, is a simple schematic of the cognitive, neurochemical, behavioral, and emotional "process of change" that occurs as we think.

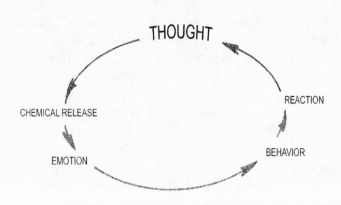

Thought Cycle

Over the life-span, our thoughts vary in their degrees of development and clarity. Our thoughts release chemicals in the brain that, neurochemically, produce emotions; the emotions lead to a particular behavior or set of behaviors; and, finally, we check or monitor our reaction to what has just transpired in the cycle. The Thought Cycle occurs in less than a nanosecond; then, we are "off to the races," again.

80

In other words, if we wait until we <u>feel</u> like it, we may never begin a particular action, especially, one we were not sure we wanted to take in the first place. If our reaction yields a conscious assessment that the Thought Cycle engenders *good*, connects us with someone, something, our sacred inner self, or the "other," and, basically, offers a more positive experience, then we are inclined to reinforce the thought which began the cycle. If our reaction to what the cycle produced or elicited is negative (maintains a seemingly-safe or closed place within us, such as protection from a fear that feels like a positive outcome or occurs in a negative situation), then we are inclined not to repeat that Thought Cycle. The *healthier* self moves quickly to positive thoughts, engendering healthier feelings and behaviors.

In psychotherapy, I call this the "Y-Solution," teaching the Thought Cycle and the "Y-Solution" to my clients so they can choose to be accountable, to affect actual, mentally healthy, soul-directed outcomes in any circumstance. Using the "Y-Solution," itself, fosters and reinforces clear, responsible, loving choice within everyday experience. In the Jewish expression of naming the Lord, a capital "Y" begins "YHWH" of the Name (regarded as too sacred to be pronounced). There are many exquisite words in the Hebrew and Greek languages that name God (*Adonai* meaning "Lord" or *Elohim* meaning "God" or *Kyrios* meaning "Lord") and represent the relationship of God with us.

The "Y-Solution" is very simple:

> 1)   Determine *handedness*: your dominant hand is the one you use most often to apprehend your world: to brush your teeth, to drink a class of water, and to pick up your car keys or a pencil.

> 2)   *Breathe*: as you *in*hale, push your tummy *out*, little-by-little, as far as you can (this is yoga breathing and requires practice) while gradually envisioning fresh oxygen at the upper, posterior part of your brain. As you exhale while pushing your tummy out further (yes, it is possible), envision your

81

non-dominant hand with its first two digits or fingers
held in a "Y" position; move the first finger of your
dominant hand toward the left if you are left-handed
or toward the right if you are right-handed (see the
drawings, below). If you are ambidextrous, choose
one hand to practice using the "Y-Solution" to
rethink your apprehension of the world. As you
breathe and practice the "Y-Solution" a *few* times,
you create a nearly automatic, mind's-eye visual of
its corrective thinking assistance, available instantly.

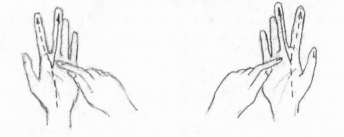

Right-handed person   Left-handed person

Breathing as in the manner and practice of ancient yoga, is a
form of biofeedback, and it is a very healthy way of breathing.
As you inhale while pushing your belly outward and taking in
fresh oxygen, two things occur: a) every organ, thus, hopefully,
each cell in your body is absorbing fresh oxygen to re-
oxygenate your blood; and, b) the hippocampus is claiming its
nanosecond override that *all is well*, thus interrupting the "fight
or flight" message of the amygdala. An even flow of oxygen-
rich blood circulates without fits of stop/start, so the amygdala's
fear response is not being triggered to do its age-old and
otherwise necessary job in the limbic system.

3) *Rethink* (see the Thought Cycle, p. 80): the "Y-Solution"
   requires a conscious <u>choice</u>. Deep within the brain, we
   are relearning and retraining our innate, biological
   response to anger, resentment, hurt, and fear; we are
   able to do so because we are safe, knowing and

experiencing the consciousness of thought-full peace within ourselves. We have just breathed fresh oxygen to support our mental alertness, and we are consciously present, guided by this inner clarity and strength to choose a well direction. As clients leave my office, I encourage them, saying, "Stay in a well direction."

As you become more practiced in using the "Y-Solution," you may choose to add a deeply spiritual step during the process of exhaling and rethinking. In the beginning and when you are in a setting to permit the movement, relax your arms and place your hands on your knees, palms up and open when sitting or, if standing, anywhere, allow your arms to fall easily and gently by your sides. *As you exhale and rethink (tummy relaxed), speak and breathe the word "ru-ah" which means Spirit or Holy Spirit in ancient Greek.* What begins to happen is that you will not need to use the *handed* motion because you will envision the directional shift instantly in your mind, and you will not need to say ru-ah; it, also, will be in your brain and new thoughts.

The "Y-Solution" works because the cognitive retraining, our relearning, is taking place in the brain, in the mind's thoughts, again, in the power of the Holy Spirit. Jesus tells us, in Luke 17:21, the kingdom of God is within. We breathe, in the present moment, with our healthier thoughts resulting in healthier emotions and actions. The neurological plasticity of the brain produces new levels of growth and development. A positive thinking process -- an honest, blessed way of feeling, behaving, and evaluating our newly thought choice creates wellness, one day at a time. *Staying in a well direction* continually creates opportunities for healthier life.

It is the purpose and effect of the second letter in the GBU process to make conscious our healing self. Gradually, we *learn to hope in the continuance of* the neurologically real, spiritual, and developmental *dying to self* as we are given to create new life.

Beginning Life Anew

Chapter Five

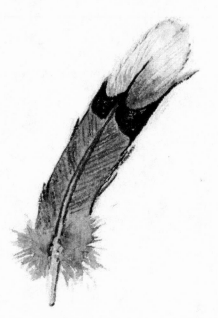

As a new plant breaks the ground with great difficulty. . .so must we sometimes push against difficulty in bringing forth our dreams.

From the *I Ching*: Hexagram #3 "Chaos"

Beginning Life Anew

Chapter Five

The Second of Two in the GBU Letters

To recap, the second letter is to be written *only after three whole days have passed following* the burning of the first GBU letter. The three-day period means a consecutive 72 hours or greater after the burning of the first letter. You can write the second letter on the fourth day, or the 10th day, or the 80th day, or any number of days after the 72-hour timeframe has passed. Only one, first, GBU letter and its companion second letter are to be written at a time. If you want or need to write a first GBU letter to more than one person or other loss, it is very important to complete the pair of letters: the first GBU letter followed, at least three days later, by your writing of its companion second letter to yourself from the person, pet or other loss *before* you begin another first GBU letter.

It is vital to understand that the second letter opens the way for God to bring blessings, God's purpose, and deep, true, sacred, and joyous gifts to you from the full experience of the loss. You may think there are no blessings in your loss. In 2 Chronicles 30:1, we read of how Hezekiah, king of Judah, encourages all of Israel and Judah, also sending letters to Ephraim and Manasseh, calling them to keep the Passover in Jerusalem in the house of the Lord:

> "O People of Israel, return to the Lord, the God of Abraham, Isaac, and Israel, that he may turn again to the remnant of you who have escaped from the hand of the kings of Assyria. Do not be like your fathers and your brethren, who were faithless to the Lord God of their fathers, so that he made them a desolation, as you see.

87

Do not now be stiff-necked as your fathers were, but yield yourselves to the Lord, and come to his sanctuary, which he has sanctified for ever, and serve the Lord your God, that his fierce anger may turn away from you. For if you return to the Lord, your brethren and your children will find compassion with their captors, and return to this land. For the Lord your God is gracious and merciful, and will not turn away his face from you, if you return to him." . . . For there were many in the assembly who had not sanctified themselves; therefore the Levites had to kill the passover lamb for every one who was not clean, to make it holy to the Lord. For a multitude of the people, many of them from Ephraim, Manasseh, Issachar, and Zebulun, had not cleansed themselves, yet they ate the passover otherwise than as prescribed. For Hezekiah had prayed for them, saying, "The good Lord pardon every one who sets his heart to seek God, the Lord the God of his fathers, even though not according to the sanctuary's rules of cleanness." And the Lord heard Hezekiah, and healed the people. And the people of Israel that were present at Jerusalem kept the feast of unleavened bread seven days with great gladness; and the Levites and the priests praised the Lord day by day, singing with all their might to the Lord. And Hezekiah spoke encouragingly to all the Levites who showed good skill in the service of the Lord. So the people ate the food of the festival for seven days, sacrificing peace offerings and giving thanks to the Lord the God of their fathers.[1]

We read the Lord revealing God in this beautiful call to us and in the Lord God's gift of sanctifying healing.

A reminder: the second of the two GBU letters is the one you write to yourself. The second letter yields love and forgiveness from your soul, from God, from all that is holy. When you seek the Lord's guidance in writing the second letter, you will be humbled and delighted in knowing the presence of the Holy Spirit in bringing forth God's gifts to you from the loss. The process that is fruitful and healing is to write the words you need to hear, you need to read, whether or not the person (if the letter is from a person) would have used the same words. There are no columns in the second letter; a standard format is suggested.

Many second letters begin, "Dear <u>your name</u>, I love you. I am sorry. . . for dying, for leaving you, for never having met you, for never having had a relationship with you, for no longer being there in-person to laugh, love, grocery shop, play ball with you, bake cookies with you, watch you grow up, watch the children and grandchildren grow up, enjoy retirement with you, hold you, love you, help you extinguish the candles on your birthday cake, make sushi with or for you, dry your tears." The letter then continues with other feelings or thoughts: "I was wrong to, I wish we had, no one else ever shared 'that' with me but you, and I shall be in your heart when you . . . . Please forgive me. I love you. I am with you, always." When you experience relationship with the loss as hurtful, your closing to the second letter may be more formal or it may be simply a name.

Even the profoundly healing chemicals in tears no longer will be needed, once the deeper healing is known to you, its gifts a part of your very soul. Even though we may carry our grieving, it is a life choice, a gift to your mind, your body, and your soul when you embrace writing *both* letters, yielding deep healing of present or long-ago loss. Paul tells us, "For godly grief produces a repentance that leads to salvation and brings no regret, but worldly grief produces death."[2]

The second letter can be as brief or as lengthy as you choose. What matters *most* in the second letter is the presence and fullness of love expressed to you or humble atonement from a person you did not like or want to forgive. You can choose to keep the second letter, forever, or you may be creative in what you do with it when you no longer need to read it. While you retain the letter, seal it in an envelope; then, each time you take it out and read it, place the letter back in the first envelope, and place that envelope in a second envelope. You may end up with one envelope or many envelopes, nested, one in another.

Delaying or Not Writing the Second Letter

We can postpone writing the second letter or not write it at all, choosing to forget about it in our desire to move forward and (even) to write another first GBU letter to someone else. When we delay or do not write the second letter, it is likely something else is going on within us. We might think if we complete the process of writing the second letter, we would lose our connection to the very person, pet, life event or material loss from whom or which we do not want to separate. In grieving, the anxiety of separating or relinquishing the fear of separation from the loss can seem overwhelming and downright scary. The conscious choice, itself, to write the second letter changes the brain. Our unconscious, unbeknownst to us, also is taking care of us; it will yield core healing. When we become aware that we do not want to write the second letter or we simply cannot find the time to do so, we can take a positive step by exploring several questions.

Do we struggle to forgive ourselves? This age-old question reaches the heart of healing loss. Why is this struggle true for us? As we mature, we learn we are more alike as whole persons, than different. At times, such realization is an eye-opener and it is one we do not acknowledge easily. Our insight calls us to be humble and to forgive; we move closer to *getting back in the river*. Our conscious growth is in recognition of each soul's need to love and to be loved; thereby, we invite, encourage, and honor the sacred within one another, in our relationship with the God of our understanding, and, as St. Augustine stated, in our desire to "respect the dignity of each person." The latter we may know as *The Golden Rule*: "Do unto others as you would have them do unto you;" or, as the Second Commandment: "Love your neighbor as yourself."

Sometimes, we forget to be kind to ourselves even though we are kind to others. The process of forgiveness opens the way for us to recognize ourselves in the experiences of other people: we empathize with them to varying degrees of hurt from and fear of separation, from ourselves, from one another, from God, all that is sacred. In the act of forgiving, we move through our next *dying to self*; we reach another and deeper level of sacred self-acceptance, making it possible to remain open in our acceptance of another person. Each time we forgive one another and offer acceptance, we are being love and we are at-peace; the only way to know the truth of these words is to forgive.

An equally vital question remains, "Are we afraid to trust God?" In the deep pain of loss, perhaps, still angry with God, a person, a pet or an event that changed our lives, yet, seeking healing, we can begin to recognize and acknowledge this question in our quiet, innermost thoughts and feelings. We could continue to anthropomorphize God, making God in our image (see p. 18). What if we have not written the second letter due to a certainty in our belief that the person or loss would not forgive us? Maybe, we have felt the pain of hurt, anger, separation, or depression for such a long time that we cannot see ourselves living without those feelings. Might we "prefer" to feel somewhat empty inside or to remain angry, rather than to feel the depth of those feelings? At least anger brings passions of its own, even if such passions are not the full living of life that seemed to leave, utterly disappear, when we experienced the loss. We are totally unaware of a deeper fear: if we complete the grieving process, we are afraid we will lose the person, forever. At this point, we do not know we are protecting ourselves with a continually toxic outcome; and, we have interrupted our grieving.

Our unconscious *is working* to bring us healing. Protecting ourselves from what feels like further loss appears to be easier than entering the whole set of seemingly complex thoughts and emotions related to our grief. It is true: we *will* cope at all costs. Our tenacity is understandable; yet, only a fraction of the depth *in living and accepting the gift in the death, the loss or dying to self, in the meaning of life* can be known. Not grieving the loss has consequences. Not grieving stunts our growth in all aspects of our being: spiritual, cognitive, emotional, interpersonal, and physical. When we do not grieve, we cannot continue to evolve and develop our sacred self, who we are as whole beings, evolving in grace, within ourselves, with one another, *with* God. Writing another *first* GBU letter, *before* we finish the second of the two letters about the same loss, serves to reinforce our minimal awareness of (if we are, at all, open and receptive), or disbelief in the beautiful gifts of God intrinsic to the loss. We cannot know the awaiting depth of healing. The second letter beckons to be written; sacred gifts of the heart invite healing.

When we no longer need to read the second letter, we will know it. The depth and truth of the forgiveness in the loss, within ourselves, will be complete, will be healed. One simple example of recognizing the place of healing is to take out our high school yearbook and read one of those long messages from a close friend; we begin to realize we know its contents and we can proceed to read another page or long note. At this point, we have *introjected* (unconsciously accepted) the loving message in our yearbook. The same introjection is operating, at some point and at multiple levels of awareness, when we read and reread the second letter written to us from the loss; we are reading its truth and receiving it. Profound depths of understanding and forgiveness result from introjecting the gifts in the second letter; such is the purity of soul-knowing.

Now, we can choose to tie a ribbon of yellow, or red, or white, or emerald, or pink, or indigo, or orange, or purple, or silver, or gold, or any combination of colors of ribbons around the second letter and place it in a secure place. We can choose to do something else with our second letter. For example, we may place the letter under the root-ball of a new tree, or place the second letter beneath a new rose bush, hydrangea or forsythia, or any other plant. If we live near a body of water, the ocean, a pond or brook, river, stream, lake, canal, or waterfall, and, for those taking small steps to protect the environment, if we have thought ahead and written the second letter on biodegradable paper, we can shred the letter and throw the pieces of paper in the water (all shall be healed, "*all shall be well*"), or burn the letter and throw the ashes in the water, or place the ashes under a new tree or plant.[3] Anything creative and beautiful is appropriate.

Our task is to accept graciously the love offered and present in the loss, to introject the *depth of healing* intrinsic to its gifts, and to *embrace its learnings*. The gifts are genuine and our call *is to accept* the deepest love from the loss which we would have accepted at an earlier time, if the loss had been able to communicate its sacredness in our life. Jesus, the Logos, calls us to be at-peace, and walks with us, overcoming the world. Hence, in the grace and power of the Holy Spirit, we are one with God and with our loved one or other gift in the former loss. In Philippians, Paul tells us:

> But whatever gain I had, I counted as loss for the sake of Christ. Indeed I count everything as loss because of the surpassing worth of knowing Christ Jesus my Lord. For his sake I have suffered the loss of all things, and count them as refuse, in order that I may gain Christ and be found in him, not having a righteousness of my own, based on law, but that which is through faith in Christ, the righteousness from God that depends on faith; that I may know him and the power of his resurrection, and may share his sufferings, becoming like him in his death, that if possible I may attain the resurrection from the dead.[4]

If you are struggling with the decision to write the second letter, go to a quiet place and write an addendum to the first (GBU) letter. This time, write only a third column in the GBU letter, the *uglies*; be open and honest, hold nothing back. Utterly deplete the toxic thoughts and feelings you are keeping in your less-conscious mind. Invite healing, encourage yourself to remain present, to remember, and to be kind to yourself, for you did not *know* you were withholding toxic content; otherwise, you would have released it. Remember, the *hand*-writing of the GBU letters, inclusive of releasing the worst-of-the-worst, hurtful thoughts and feelings in the *uglies* column, itself, changes your brain as you let them go, surrendering them to a healthier, more sacredly-present you. Once you have completed your addendum to the GBU letter, burn it; wait three days (72 hours or longer), and you shall be ready to write the second letter, able to embrace the love it offers.

The three-day hiatus between burning the first GBU letter and writing the second letter is a waiting period based upon the three days following the death of Jesus on the cross and his resurrection. All of life as we have known it prior to this time has died, changed forever. With the Lord, we begin again in the moment, in the eternal now, as Henri Nouwen observed.

Even seemingly brief, agonizing at times, mundane at others, impossible for us to fathom moments, days, and indescribable points in time will bring new learning as we surrender our fear and lives to God. We shall continue to heal in dreams (known to us or not), and in *core healing* resulting from the deep processing of hurtful loss. As we relax, truly trust God with us, use ancient yoga breathing, apply the Thought Cycle and the "Y-Solution," healthier cells are emerging in our mind and body. Every cell is releasing toxins and our body is releasing tensions. Our brain, mind, and emotions continue to heal, guided by the Holy Spirit's clarity of love and forgiveness. It is difficult, if not truly impossible, to go back to a less-well self. The healthy thoughts and behaviors create a much truer, present, and blessed -- that we may be a blessing to others -- sacred self evolving in the heart of God. Our inner peace will be real, more constant and immediate, grounded in healing grace and forgiveness, the love of God.

Beginning Life Anew

Sample First GBU Letter

Format of the first GBU letter

Dear *Mom* (or other person, pet, event, dream),

Good	*Bad*	*Uglies*
You loved us and you love us, now.	You died too soon; I was 12.	I didn't get to say I love you before you went into a coma.
I look like you.	I look like you.	After our disagreement about the school trip, I told you I hated you. I don't want these feelings.
I love you.	You're not here.	I hate you for dying!
Dad is here for us.	He isn't you, Mom.	He is working so hard to help us, yet, he is grieving, too.
I love Dad, too.	I don't want HIS help!	He is the one who was driving and you are the one who died. I hate him for living. Aaghh!

Sample Second Letter

Dear Name/Endearment (e.g., the "child" who composed the letter to Mom, above),

I love you! Please forgive me for dying when you were not *ready*. I think it is delightful that we look alike. There is only one you, my dear *child's name*, and you have much to give. While you may be upset with me, now, I shall be with you

95

always, and more nearly, and more dearly as you continue to heal. Dad is not responsible for my death. The van came out of nowhere and hit us. He loves you dearly, too, and is so present to help you in any way. . . .

Love, forever, my dear, sweet *child's name*,

Mom

Beginning Life Anew

Chapter Six

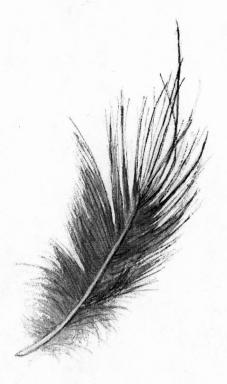

You are healed of a suffering only by experiencing it to the full.

Marcel Proust

Beginning Life Anew

Chapter Six

Joining the Healing

The verb, "to heal," means: to make sound or whole; to restore to health; to cause an undesirable condition to be overcome; to mend; to patch up a breach or division; to restore to original purity or integrity; and, in the intransitive verb form, to return to a sound state. The synonym given is "cure."[1] Dr. William C. Menninger, a founder of The Menninger Clinic in Topeka, Kansas, identified seven criteria indicative of an emotionally mature person:

1) An ability to deal constructively with reality;

2) The capacity to adapt to change;

3) A relative freedom from symptoms that are produced by tensions and anxieties;

4) The capacity to find more satisfaction in giving than receiving;

5) The capacity to relate to other people in a consistent manner with mutual satisfaction and helpfulness;

6) The capacity to sublimate, to direct one's instinctive hostile energy into creative and constructive outlets; and,

7) The capacity to love.[2]

Health care journals are replete with studies evidencing statistically significant healing when our medical and/or mental health providers treat various presenting illnesses following established protocols, and deliver care with attention, kindness, and respect. Physicians and psychotherapists acknowledge far more often, today, a deep connection with their own faith traditions and more readily encourage patients to develop spiritual health, as well. William, Abbot of St. Thierry (ca. 1085-1148), speaks of three states of spiritual growth and our progress in them: the animal state, concerned with the body; the rational state, concerned with the soul; and, the spiritual state, where we find rest only in God. It is the Holy Spirit who guides us in each state of growth.[3] We can share our steps along the way and, respectfully, offer positive thoughts, prayer, and a myriad of other loving actions.

When our relationships are based on mutual respect, lived in kindness and with nurturing honesty, we are love, one with God and one another, we are living in grace. "The only way we can come into union with God is through love."[4] Each of us is a part of one another: what happens to one of us, to any part of life, happens to all of us in some manner or form. Joining our deepest healing is to forgive, to love fully, living in the Logos, the Word and heart of God. Love calls us to walk in faith, to know one another, to be known fully, and to unite with each other in all goodness, no matter how often we err. It is to walk more nearly in forgiveness, connect in loving action, and to be thankful for the faithfulness and grace of God.

Faith is life, and it is the gift of the Lord God, the work of the Holy Spirit overflowing in grace and mercy. As M. Basil Pennington says of William of St. Thierry, "The way of faith leads to being fully integrated into the inner life of the Trinity by an affective (emotion) union with the Holy Spirit, who is the communion of the Father and the Son. This is brought about by what William calls illuminating grace, a grace which brings faith beyond intellectual understanding to the intuitive experiential knowledge and understanding that comes from love-experience of the Beloved."[5] Pennington continues by saying that William's teaching is ever present in his writings, clearly suggesting William lived this relationship, and that it shaped and guided his "outlook on life as a spiritual journey, a journey into God."[6]

It is the Lord, the work of the Holy Spirit in our lives who creates openness, respect, and acceptance within us. In *truth,* without God's presence in us, the *living out or walk* and making present qualities of healthy relationship would be more than very-difficult-at-times for us, it would be impossible. Grace and mercy abound; we *are* the Lord's Beloved. Thanks be to God.

When we seek the God of our understanding in mutual respect, our presence becomes clearer: we offer agape, unconditional love, genuine acceptance of one another, and an experience and a reflection of grace. We can meet another person who lives an "other" way of life, quite different from our own, uniting *inspiritus*, teaching and learning in communion with the sacred. During the years of her extensive ministry, it was said of Mother Teresa of Calcutta that her life was her prayer. In*deed*, it matters that we laugh, cry, touch, and think, pray, love, and live as well as is possible every day. We are created to glorify God, *to love the Christ in one another; we do so in each life-calling when we grow and evolve in the power and fellowship of the Holy Spirit.* Every time we accept that call, in each moment, we are *getting back in the river*.

When we choose to write the first GBU letter, honestly and completely, holding nothing back in the *releasing* of hurtful thoughts or stored memories, even if the loss represented so much good and our expression is one of the *sadness of missing*, then we are open to joining the healing present in the second letter. The mystical presence of God who suffers with us and eternally brooks every seeming obstacle, brings us loving peace and returns the full truth of the loss relationship, in love, to our hearts. Our life is to honor God's love; our joy is to give it away.

We Heal the Past in the Present

We heal the past in the present; it is the only time we have to live and to seek eternal life. Over seventeen years ago, a client who had been among the ground-troops as an armed soldier in an earlier war, sought help for depression, overtly presenting in overwhelming rage that he had medicated for years with varying forms of substance abuse. Nearing mid-life, the man was ready to grow, and accepted the hospital program entrance and participation requirements of complete abstinence from substance use. We spent a year meeting three times per week in individual psychotherapy sessions during which time my client also participated in a variety of hospital-based groups on topics covering dozens of unfamiliar and unexpressed feelings. In painfully emerging health, my client shared his thoughts about his role and actions in the war. At first, this man expressed only feelings of anger and sadness (the child within himself) about his family of origin, and the loss of hope that he would ever return to healthy life, coupled with his deep desire to do so. This man's story was tragic and not unusual in the loss of himself. When my client was eight years old, he and his seven year-old brother were walking home from school. As the boys approached their home, the police were walking out of the house, pushing a gurney with a body-bag resting on it; their father, in handcuffs, followed the gurney. With no explanation about the incident, the police officers drove the boys to the home of a family member. Their mother was the person in the body-bag; their father had killed her, was convicted, and, subsequently, spent twenty years in prison.

During the last ten of those same twenty years, my client had served in the war. As we worked together, I encouraged my client to create drawings representing his feelings. We met for several months before he felt safe enough to do any art therapy with me. Finally, he began, drawing only black everything: circles, jagged lines, clouds, squiggles, all too dense with darkness to discern when each drawing was complete. At some point, he broke through his repressed feelings of anger, hurt, and fear, and sobbed for a long time. He was able to write the contents of the first GBU letter, no longer afraid of the *uglies* hiding in the dark. Initially, he could remember only "the first kill," an expression I heard later from other war vets. Through the early years following their father's release from prison, this man had remained connected with his younger brother; my client had not seen their father. In his sixth or seventh month of therapy, I asked my client if he would consider inviting his brother and father to the hospital program's monthly family night; he declined to think about it. We kept working together. Two months after the suggestion, my client arrived and stood in the doorway of my office, saying that his father and brother would be coming to family night, and asking if I would please be available to meet them? YES.

In time, my client was able to share with his father his deep hurt in the loss of his mother and his feelings about the violent manner in which her death had occurred. My client spoke of healing his formerly unrecognized need to repress his own previous behaviors, even though sanctioned by a war *in order to* become like his father and *to obtain his father's approval*; otherwise, he would have continued to repress his hatred of the action of murder which he had committed, also. He shared his absence of verifiable information about his mother's lack of self-defense (an entirely other set of inner and interpersonal work); and, that he wanted to begin life anew. This man was blessed to hear from his father the deep contents of the companion second letter and to write them. Not every story contains such hurtful behaviors; yet, many stories identify the need for core healing and life anew, as represented in this client's losses of mother, father, family life, "killings" of persons, and himself.

As my client, above, experienced, *joining the healing* that emerges from completing the GBU letters is a vital gift we can choose to give ourselves. Deep healing flows from courageous exploration of the degradation of life that may have resulted from unresolved grief. We *know*, a mind and spirit knowing, often a soma or body knowing, that something is very different, now. Our deep knowing is a paradigm shift within: we are clearer, lighter, and healed of hurtful, tearful, and debilitating inner tugs that used to keep us out of the river, not fully participating in life. Increasingly, we become aware that this difference already has occurred; now, it is in the past. This time, there is no guilt for not seeing a face or not remembering a voice; in its place, joy and laughter, a new, real, nearly unspeakable truth-in-connecting with other people because the love inherent in the gift of the loss *is* a healed part of our soul. Our energy returns, with or without medication, as may be medically warranted. We begin to notice the deep inner shift has occurred and continues with less of a conscious effort on our part. We are graced with humble awareness of the Holy Spirit's presence and power within; and, yes, life will continue to challenge us to grow and evolve. Thanks be to God.

If you have written the first GBU letter and you are not experiencing this "lightness of being" concerning your loss, perhaps, you were not fully forthcoming in the *uglies* section of the letter. Remember, the best step is to be totally honest with yourself and to write an addendum to the first letter; you do not need to recreate the entire first GBU letter. You will know if your release of additional *uglies* brings deep healing by the presence of loving expression *to you*, in the addition to your second letter about the same loss. A minister once said in a sermon that God asks three things of us: one, to be kind; two, to be kind; and, three, to be kind.

We, being united in our healing with the blessings of the loss, now are far more kind with others, also. Our soul continues to teach us, and our learning to be kind from the holiness within begins to yield *ripples of loving action* going out to others.

> Thou dost keep him in perfect peace, whose mind is stayed on thee, because he trusts in thee.[7]

Beginning Life Anew

Chapter Seven

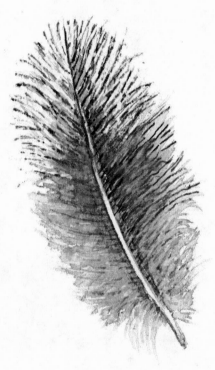

Thy way, O God, is holy.

Psalm 77:13

Beginning Life Anew

Chapter Seven

Transcending the Pain of Loss is Real

As we accept the loss and its inherent *dying to self* in our walk with the Lord, we are healing in the grace and power of the Holy Spirit. Ancient theology texts remind us: when we transcend the pain of our loss we are transformed. Basil Pennington encourages us to embrace the teachings of William of St. Thierry: 'Yet even for the beginner, William dares to trace out the full meaning of transforming union, *unitas spiritus,* union of spirit with God, "for to see God . . . is faith's proper desire." It is by love, the sense of the soul, that we are transformed into what we love, not in nature but in affection. But in this life God can only be perceived "as in a riddle." So we depend on the understanding that comes from above, the action of the gifts of the Holy Spirit.'[1]

God meets us in prayer, in tears, and in music, all of which create deep healing and inspiration. "Weeping is one of the best forms of prayer," offers Father Mark Delery, former Abbot of Holy Cross Abbey in Berryville, Virginia, priest and author, and physician for over 50 years.[2] Beautiful music uplifts, resonating in the soul as a quiet tone or as a complete symphony of chords and *dis*chords, beautiful and hurtful, all sacred and healed through life. And so we learn of God: love, present in the letting go and in the embracing of gifts of the loss, continues to ripple out, returning and uniting us with all that is holy.

With a clear mind and heart, we reach new, real depths of understanding and trust, known to us as pure holiness, grace and mercy. We have walked into the valley of loss and despair, what I call *the wolf cry in the night* (certain we would be annihilated), in the presence of all that is sacred, the *good*, the *bad*, and the *uglies*. This time we are not in *the Jell-O pool*. We know God is with us and with our loved ones, and we are *united in being* with them, deep within our heart and soul where only love lives. Now, in pure grace, with much prayer and *sacred* homework, we are *getting back in the river*. What comes to mind is the knowledge that it takes 12-to-18 months to move through the early, deep healing of loss that occurs only when we attend to our grieving, and remain open to the love of God in so many quiet, painful, and glorious moments of grace and forgiveness.

As we work through our grieving, the change we experience is a transcendence of the pain in or to which we were *stuck* (see Chapter Four). Transcending the pain of our loss, the experience of sacredness in *releasing* and healing, of walking through our pain and sometimes feeling as though we are crawling through our pain, brings about our inner transformation, helping us with openness to acknowledge the eternal truth contained in the loss. Trusting God with us, in grace, we have peeled away layers of seeming-protection; in deep healing, also in grace, we embrace as a blessing our inner work and its sacred gifts. Often, the most challenging aspect of writing the GBU letters is to *rethink* "what we think of as" *transcendence*: many people articulate their understanding of the concept of transcendence to be that of moving on, giving in or being free of something or someone. We hear the hurtful phrase, "just get over it," when a person has not known healing, the sacred working-through of bereavement. Transcendence, the quality or state of being transcendent, is recognized as exceeding the limits of ordinary understanding, experience or knowledge, even being beyond comprehension or surpassing material existence or the universe. It is interesting to ponder what may be a very close link between transcendence and the (or a) function of the epigenome; why would we be surprised? After all, we are created in the image of God.

Deep healing and genuine growth result when we work through the grieving process, using the GBU letters as a vehicle for change. Our change is a transcendence of the pain, our negative attachment or fear of separation. Aware or not, we were *stuck*. Less an understanding and more an *experience of transcendence* with regard to the GBU letters, suggests that holy immanence, within us, **is** such that we join, incorporate, and even become, while never exhausting the depths of, Sacred, loving, and forgiving relationship. We are lifted up in the holy, loving arms of our Lord. Transcendence brings transformation and blessing; we are, in holiness, in a true and mystical way, one with the gifts of the loss, and we experience pure, total, and eternal, inner peace. If you do not know this peace, with or without an awareness of needing to heal a loss, please be encouraged to continue to seek God who is faithful, unconditionally loves us, and is only eternal healing and joy.

Celebrating the Sacred of God

God lives in community and calls us to do the same: when we love freely, genuinely, we have only begun to accept another person. Just as the depth of understanding or other-person knowledge is infinite, so is it eternal and grace-filled. Since love is of God and cannot be un-love, so is it immaterial and a mere infinitesimal reflection of the Holy. Each of us knows the sacred in life cannot be explained, cannot be denied and truly never ends, and is pure, quintessential joy, love, mercy, and forgiveness. God is *humbling and inviting, faith and forgiveness in love* in an instant, in a tone of voice, in a laughter-filled moment or a smile only deep love can share. Our true being in grace, the ***altar of kindness*** in our midst is God, the Sacred Spirit of love.[3]

In grace *we are blessed* to live and breathe love every day. We are called, daily, over and over and over, again, to higher and deeper and wider breadths of God, to celebrate joyously, humbly, and fully the grace-to-become, and to meet the imago in one another. In this way we transcend death, our *dying to self* creates new life and we are alive in the eternal Holy Spirit of God. Our transformation in grace, evolving and becoming who we are created to be, is a process in which we are teaching and learning together, creating new depths of affection by being love in truth: *how* (as is expressed in faith traditions around the world) God *is* love.

In his exquisite, three-hour, quiet film, *Into Great Silence*, Philip Gröning gives us the privilege of living with a group of Carthusian Monks in the Grande Chartreuse, a 12th Century monastery in the French Alps.[4] These monks are known to be among the most ascetic in the world. Season-to-season, they live quiet, humble, joyous, and visibly unchanging lives. Their world is beautiful, seemingly simple in its day-by-day challenge to grow and meet God in Christ, in one another, and in every task and mode in community, enriched and blessed beyond words. God reveals and is revealed in every action, in each personality, life of prayer, and shared responsibility.

Whether an artist, engineer, parent, farmer, night-rider keeping the city clean, priest or poet, everything is different when we humbly walk in joyous relationship with God. This *is* sacred faithfulness. God *is* holy, *is* with us, Emmanuel, in and through everything, calling us to do and be the same with each other: in kindness of truth, with faithful perseverance, in the steadfast love of Christ exemplified by the Cross. In The School of Charity, Evelyn Underhill speaks her understanding of these truths:

> A Christian's belief about reality is a wonderful blend of confidence and experience. On one hand it asks great faith in the invisible . . . on the other hand it includes and embraces the hardest facts of the actual life we know and gives them a creative quality. It is a religion which leaves nothing out. The Word, the Thought of God, made flesh and dwelling among us, accepted our conditions, did not impose His. It is as complete human beings, taught and led by a complete Humanity, that we respond to the pressure of God. There are other forms of saving tribulation than martyrdom, many ways of enduring to the end; but none that does not involve the painful conflict between softness and sturdiness, natural self-love and supernatural divine love. Grace does not work *in vacuo*: it works on the whole man, that many-levelled creature; and shows its perfect work in One who is described as Very Man, and of whom we cannot think without the conflict of Gethsemane and the surrender of the Cross. Suffering has its place within the Divine purpose, and is transfigured by the touch of God. A desperate crisis, the demand for a total self-giving, a

110

willingness to risk everything, an apparent failure, darkness and death – all these are likely to be incidents of a spiritual course. . . . examine [our] . . . capacity for suffering and love. [In the New Testament] we find a suffering and love twined so closely together, that we cannot wrench them apart: and if we try to do so, the love is maimed in the process – loses its creative power – and the suffering remains, but without its aureole of willing sacrifice.[5]

The steadfastness of God's love is our living example, one that can be our chosen action with one another. "Profound submission to the Will of God declared through circumstances: being what we are, and the world what it is, that means sooner or later Gethsemane, and the Cross, and the darkness of the Cross. Most of the saints have been through that. We do not begin to understand the strange power of the Passion, the light it casts on existence, till we see what it was in their lives. For union with the Cross means experience of the dread fact of human nature, that only those who are willing to accept suffering up to the limit are capable of giving love up to the limit; and that this is the only kind of love which can be used for the purposes of the redeeming life."[6]

How can we bring these two realities of connection together, what we live of holy love and our experience of suffering in darkness, the fear of life's places of abandonment, particularly, when we have known a significant death or loss? God is with us through everything. As we yield our fear *to* love, *to* God, and little-by-little learn to trust the gentle, calm voice within us, we find our lives truly changing, we are living in grace. Such is James Fowler's sixth and highest level of living, *where being and doing are one.*[7] According to quantum physicists, we live in multiple dimensions of reality, perhaps, as many as eleven. Within ourselves, we are empowered to live indwelled by the Holy Spirit, *with* God. The steadfast love and faithfulness of God are eternal, *inspiritus*, breathing in and through all to reach us, in a moment, at any moment, and in *be*ing with one another, calling upon our inner strength to be love. The Lord will not lose one of us. The Holy Spirit will use everything and go to any length to let us know God walks with us, forgives us, heals us, and loves us, unconditionally, forever.

The GBU letters are meaning-full and highly focused vehicles to help us reach previously unconscious, and, otherwise, consciously inaccessible thoughts and feelings, those which are imperative to the mind, body, Spirit healing of loss. Our hearts are given the grace to become whole again. Most of us take awhile to learn or to relearn how to paddle or swim or float in the river. Keep learning. Keep seeking the sacred: the love of God.

The GBU letters are unique, distinct, opening the way to *getting back in the river*. You are a blessing. Please remember, joy is true, deep, real. Be encouraged. In our walk with the Lord, and in the eternal purpose of God, the Holy Spirit is beginning life anew within each of us and continues to bless our healing. In Revelation (7:13-17) we read:

> Then one of the elders addressed me, saying, "Who are these, clothed in white robes, and whence have they come?" I said to him, "Sir, you know." And he said to me, "These are they who have come out of the great tribulation; they have washed their robes and made them white in the blood of the Lamb. Therefore are they before the throne of God, and serve him day and night within his temple; and he who sits upon the throne will shelter them with his presence. They shall hunger no more, neither thirst any more; the sun shall not strike them, nor any scorching heat. For the Lamb in the midst of the throne will be their shepherd, and he will guide them to springs of living water; and God will wipe away every tear from their eyes."

Thanks be to God.

Amen

112

GETTING BACK IN THE RIVER
The GBU Letters

Beginning Life Anew

Chapter Notes and References

Unless otherwise indicated, all Scripture quotations are from
<u>The Holy Bible: Revised Standard Version</u>. New York, NY:
Thomas Nelson & Sons, Old Testament Section, 1952; New
Testament Section, 1946.

<u>Opening paragraph</u>

Doherty, Catherine de Hueck (1896-1985). <u>Molchanie:</u>
<u>Experiencing the Silence of God</u>. Combermere, Ontario,
Canada: Madonna House Publications, 2001, p. 14. *Molchanie*
is the Russian word for 'silence' (back cover). Catherine was
born into a wealthy, Russian Orthodox family and served as a
nurse during World War I., through the civil war and starvation
of the Russian Revolution. Catherine escaped to England after
1917 and moved to Canada in 1921. In Canada, she "accepted
the teachings of the Catholic Church without rejecting the
spiritual wealth of her Orthodox heritage" (p. 87), living with
and serving the poor in Harlem, New York, and in Toronto,
Canada. At the suggestion of the Archbishop of Toronto and
with the full support of her husband, Eddie, Catherine began
Friendship House to serve the poor, and those living in rural
communities in Canada and in several major U.S. cities. In
1947, Catherine established a spiritual center, Friendship House
Apostolate, now named Madonna House Apostolate, whose
training center is in Combermere, Ontario, Canada, with
foundations in eight countries, others sites in Canada, and in the
United States. The Madonna House training center "offers an
experience of Gospel life to hundreds every year" (p. 89). In
1962, just as the Second Vatican Council was to begin,

Catherine "established the West's first *poustinia* – a desert place of fasting and praying for unity in, with, and through Christ, a unity 'that could only be the fruit of love.' " Translated into several dozen languages, Catherine's book, Poustinia, was awarded the notable *Prix Goncourt* of the *Academie Francais*. Poustinia is considered to be a work that "witnesses to her spiritual depth and passionate zeal to pass on her faith in God" (p. 89). At this writing, Catherine Doherty has been given the official title, "Servant of God," and is being considered for sainthood in the Roman Catholic Church.

Chapter One

1.   Ezekiel 47:6b-9.

2.   Luther, Martin. Treasury of Daily Prayer. St. Louis, MO: Concordia Publishing House, 2008, 20 January, pp. 1134-1135. Martin Luther speaks of sacredness: "God's Word teaches us that the sacrament of baptism has three parts. The first is just natural water . . . [Baptism] is water, but there is something more which is added to it, which makes this water glorious and holy, makes it in fact the real baptism, namely: The second part, God's Word beside and with the water, which is not something we have invented or dreamed up, but is rather the Word of Christ, who said, "Go into all the world and baptize them in the name of the Father and of the Son and of the Holy Spirit" [Matt 28:19]. When these words are added to the water, then it is no longer simple water like other water, but a holy, divine, blessed water. For where the Word of God, by which he created heaven and earth and all things, is present, there God himself is present with his power and might. . . . we must not look upon the water as simply water without the Word, but rather know that the Word with and beside the water constitutes the substance of baptism, as St. Paul says clearly in Eph. 5 [:26] that Christ washed and cleansed his bride, the church, by the washing of water with the Word, which is quite a different bath and washing than that which occurs through natural water or human washing and bathing in a tub. For here, says St.

Paul, is the Word of the living God which says, I baptize you in the name of the Father and of the Son and of the Holy Spirit; in other words, here not a man, but God himself is baptizing. For when it is done in his name it is done indeed by the holy Trinity. Then there is a third part which is necessary to make it a sacrament, namely, institution or the Word which institutes and ordains baptism; for two kinds of Word must be present in order that it be a baptism. One which is spoken with the water or baptizing, the second that which orders and commands us to baptize in this way, that is, to immerse in water and to speak these words. When these two come together, namely, the command and institution to do this and the Word with the water, which is used in accord with the institution and practices and administers the same, then this is called a baptism and is a baptism.

3.   Lindemann, Erich. "Symptomatology and Management of Acute Grief." *American Journal of Psychiatry,* 101, pp. 141-148, 1944-1945.

4.   Ibid.

5.   Kübler-Ross, Elisabeth. On Death and Dying. New York, NY: Collier, 1969.

6.   Law, William. Digitized by Google, 2009. William Law, M.A., A New Edition. London: Printed by E. Justins, 1816, p. 12. "The Spirit of Prayer; Or, The Soul Rising Out of the Vanity of Time, Into the Riches of Eternity." Part II, D. [From, The First Dialogue], being several dialogues between Academicus, Rusticus, and Theophilus, at which Humanus was present. "This selling all, Academicus, is the measure of your dying to self; all of it is to be given up; it is an apostate nature, a stolen life, brought forth in rebellion against God; it is a continual departure from him. It corrupts every thing it touches; it defiles every thing it receives; it turns all the gifts and blessings of God into covetousness, partiality, pride, hatred, and envy. All these tempers are born, and bred, and nourished, in self. They have no other place to live in, no possibility of existence,

but in that creature which is fallen from a life in God, into a life in self."

7.   Matthew 22:37, 39.

8.   John 15:12.

9.   Davis, John E. Founder and CEO of *The Resource Group* in Towson, Maryland, a private, fee-for-service group practice of over 30 years, Dr. Davis is an adjunct faculty member of Rutgers University, an expert in the field of co-occurring mental health diagnoses, and a true wisdom figure, friend, and colleague. Thank you, John.

10.   Philippians 1:6.

11.   Tisdale, William A., Jr. In a meeting on Ash Wednesday, February 25, 2009, with The Reverend Dr. William Alfred Tisdale, Jr., Director of Anglican Studies and Formation, Berkeley Divinity School at Yale; we nodded in understanding, saying, "We are not God, we are not the Savior."

12.   Hosea 11:3-4.

13.   Middleton-Moz, Jane. <u>After the Tears: Reclaiming the Personal Losses of Childhood</u>. Pompano Beach, FL: Health Communications, Inc., 1986.

14.   Edwards, David, G. "Self-Hood: The Bright Future of the Gestalt." *Journal of Contemporary Psychology*, Vol. 9, No. 1, pp. 89-94, 1977.

15.   Job 1:20-22.

16.   Job 2:7-10.

17.   Job 3:1-26.

18.   Luther, op. cit., 6 February, pp. 1187-1188.

19.   Kushner, Rabbi Harold S. <u>When Bad Things Happen to Good People</u>. New York, NY: Schocken Books, Inc., 1981.

20.   Ibid.

21.   Nouwen, Henri J. M. <u>The Inner Voice of Love: A Journey Through Anguish to Freedom</u>. New York, NY: Doubleday, 1996.

22.   Psalm 65:9b-10.

23.   Kretzmann, Paul E. <u>Treasury of Daily Prayer</u>. Op. cit., Thursday, Lent 3, p. 99.

24.   Ezekiel 47:6, 9b-12.

25.   Ephesians 5:25-26.

26.   Emoto, Masaru. Trans. by Noriko Hosoyamada. The True Power of Water: Healing and Discovering Ourselves. Hillsboro, OR: Beyond Words Publishing, Inc., 2005, pp. 147-169.

27.   Ibid., p. 145.

28.   John 3:5-7.

29.   Indermark, John. "Lent 2009: Come to the Cross." Nashville, TN: Abingdon Press, 2008, p. 7.

30.   Ezekiel 36:25-28.

31.   Indermark, loc. cit.

32.   Ephesians 1:10.

33.   John 4:14.

34.   Pierce, Brian J., OP. We Walk the Path Together: Learning from Thich Nhat Hanh and Meister Eckhart. Maryknoll, NY: Orbis Books, 2005, p. 99.

35.   Pierce, loc. cit.

36.   Lutz, Thomas. Crying: The Natural and Cultural History of Tears. New York, NY: W. W. Norton & Company, Inc., 1999.

37.   Ibid., p. 90.

38.   Ibid., p. 18.

39.   Romans 8:33b-35a, 38-39.

40.   Lutz, op. cit., p. 23.

41.   Psalm 42:1-3.

42.   Lutz, op. cit., p. 25.

43.   John 16:33.

44.   Law, loc. cit. The Right Reverend Charles L. Longest, Retired Bishop Suffragan of the Episcopal Diocese of Maryland, in 1989, was the first person from whom I heard the term, *dying to self*, used to convey an understanding of deep spiritual growth in our loving surrender to the Holy Spirit. Thank you, Charlie.

45.   Gordon, Janice. The Reverend Janice Gordon, Episcopal priest in the Diocese of Maryland, often (1989-1991) used the phrase, "going on to larger life" to refer to the deceased.

46.   Hunt, Terry. With a special thank you to Dr. Terry Hunt, for an excellent continuing education seminar on the healthy expression of emotion. New York State, NY: Omega Institute, summer, 2005.

47.   Jodi. A lovely person who sought genuine wellness of mind/body/spirit, and gave me *full* permission to use the word "stuck" as an acronym of her design: *s* (s̲ome) *t* (t̲hing), *u* (yo̲u), *c* (c̲an't), *k* (k̲eep). Thank you, Jodi.

48.   Johnson, Catherine, and Ratey, John. <u>Shadow Syndromes</u>. New York, NY: Pantheon Books, 1997.

49.   Mead, Margaret. A world renown anthropologist; the reference for Mead's comment, while attributable to her, has not been located.

50.   Romans 8:35-39.

<u>Chapter Two</u>

1.   *The Good, The Bad And The Ugly*, 1966. Alberto Grimaldi Productions, S.A. Directed by Sergio Leone, starring Clint Eastwood, the film is the "last and the grandest of the *Dollars Trilogy*."

2.   James, John W., and Cherry, Frank. <u>The Grief Recovery Handbook: A Step-by-Step Program for Moving Beyond Loss</u>. New York, NY: Harper & Row, Publishers, 1988, p. 25.

3.   The three-day, 72-hour or longer period between burning the first GBU letter, and writing the second letter to yourself (as the author) from the addressee of the first letter, stems from Christian burial. In addition, the material included in the first letter, having been burned safely, will continue to be processed (in conscious and unconscious awareness) over the three-day period, and beyond.

4.   Matthew 12:38-41.

5.   Philippians 3:1a, 7-11, 12b-17.

6.   Romans 14:1, 4, 7-9.

7.   Matthew 8:13.

8.   John 14:6a. 'Jesus said to him, "I am the way, and the truth, and the life; no one comes to the Father, but by me." '
9.   Romans 8:26-32, 34b-35a.
10.   Romans 9:19-26.
11.   Kübler-Ross, loc. cit.
12.   Walls, Donald W. 2008. Arduously working through his own life events, Donald lived the experience that awareness yields 50 percent of growth concerning a *life-learning*; acknowledging or owning the deep impact and meaning of that learning in his life yielded a significant, additional degree of inner growth. The latter acknowledgement, surrendered to the Holy Spirit, truly plumbs the depths within each person creating health and peace, improbable in another way. Thank you, Donnie.
13.   James 5:13a-b, 15-16.
14.   Mayo Clinic Health Letter, Vol. 27, N1, January, 2009.
15.   Amen, Daniel G. Change Your Brain, Change Your Life. New York, NY: Three Rivers Press, 1998.
16.   Billard, Sister Ann. A dear person, encourager, and friend. Sister Bridget Sullivan, Mother General, in grace and kindness guides the group of Sisters in their order, Sisters of Mercy of Our Lady of Charity, in Charleston, South Carolina.

Chapter Three

1.   Hospice of Queen Anne's, Inc., 255 Comet Drive, Centreville, MD. Thank you, Susan Branden.

Chapter Four

1.   Numbers 14:18; Psalms 30:5a, 145:8; Joel 2:13; Colossians 3:8-11.
2.   Psalm 145:8-9. The Psalm continues, 145:10-14:
All thy works shall give thanks to thee, O Lord,
and all thy saints shall bless thee.

They shall speak of the glory of thy kingdom, and tell of thy power, to make known to the sons of men thy mighty deeds, and the glorious splendor of thy kingdom.
Thy kingdom is an everlasting kingdom,
and thy dominion endures throughout all generations.
The Lord is faithful in all his words, and gracious in all his deeds. The Lord upholds all who are falling, and raises up all who are bowed down.

3.   James 1:20-21.
4.   Hosea 11:9.
5.   Ephesians 4:30-32, 5:1-2.
6.   Matthew 6:12, 14.
7.   Luke 23:34a.
8.   Colossians 3:8-17.
9.   Philippians 1:3-7.
10.   Romans 12:2.
11.   John 16:33.
12.   LeDoux, Joseph. The Emotional Brain: The Mysterious Underpinnings of Emotional Life. New York, NY: Simon & Schuster Adult Publishing Group, 1998.
13.   Davidson, R. J., and Fox, N. "Frontal Brain Asymmetry Predicts Infants' Response to Maternal Separation." *Journal of Abnormal Psychology*, Vol. 98, 1989, pp. 127-131.
14.   Matthew 7:7-8.
15.   This chapter note honors the work of Emero Stiegman in his exquisite analytical commentary, On Loving God, by Bernard of Clairvaux [1090-1153]. *On Loving God*, Translation, Cistercian Publications Inc., 1973; An Analytical Commentary, Cistercian Publications, 1995, Kalamazoo, Michigan. The work of Cistercian Publications is made possible in part through support from Western Michigan University to The Institute of Cistercian Studies. Stiegman's Notes:
Commentary: Note 22. Philippe Delhaye, 'La conscience morale dans la doctrine de S. Bernard [1090-1153]', *Saint Bernard theologien*, 219-221, finds in Bernard a sense of moral conscience, in the tradition of Origen, enlarged to

consciousness, with a mystic dimension—the presence of God in the soul. Michael Casey, Monk of Tarrawarra, *Athirst for God: Spiritual Desire in Bernard of Clairvaux's Sermons on the Song of Songs*, CS 77 (Kalamazoo: Cistercian Publications, 1988) 319, forcefully affirms the necessity of seeing in Bernard an exploration of more than consciousness: 'There is a zone of being which is beyond consciousness, which is pre-conscious'. Casey links the unconscious to Bernard's concept of 'the human heart', where God dwells and acts.

Commentary: Note 38, is given in its entirety: "Joseph Marechal, SJ, *Studies in the Psychology of the Mystics*, trans. with an Introduction and Forward by Algar Thorold (Albany, N.Y.: Maji Books, 1964) 166-167, concludes, 'Metaphysics and Psychology teach the same lesson of fundamental humility as does Christianity'. Bernard's manner of arguing assumes this is so. A Christian sense of the self's relation to God can, then, be shown to have a rational and psychological validity."

Stiegman's preceding Commentary: Note 37, herein cited after the reference in Latin, states, "Gra 3 (SBOp 3:168.1-9) E. Rozanne Elder, 'William of Saint Thierry: Rational and Affective Spirituality', in *The Spirituality of Western Christendom*, ed. E. Rozanne Elder, CS 30 (Kalamazoo: Cistercian Publications, 1976) 85-105, observes that, unlike William [Abbot of Saint Thierry, ca. 1085-1148?], Saint Bernard never allowed the rationalism against which he struggled to threaten his acceptance of the place of reason in the spiritual life."

16.   Kirk, William J., and Rebecca B. 2007. The Kirks are a God-centered couple, each deeply loving of the other, their children and families, and so very many people. Rebecca is a 32-year staff member with a private Episcopal school in Maryland, and William is a Roman Catholic seminary-trained counselor and educator. The Kirks understand, truly live, and lovingly model, "the importance and discipline needed to be a receiver of forgiveness;" their

comments were offered in an early reading of this manuscript. Thank you, Rebecca and Bill, for everything.

17. Frankl, Viktor E. <u>Man's Search for Meaning</u>. Boston, MA: Beacon Press, 1959.

18. Swindol, Charles A. I am grateful to Chuck Swindol's radio commentaries on *agapao*, in one of his beautifully challenging and insightful programs, and always *of* God, on WRBS, 95.1 FM, in Baltimore, MD, 2009.

19. Kirk, William J. 2007.

20. Webster, Merriam. <u>The Webster Collegiate Dictionary</u>. Springfield, MA: Merriam-Webster, Inc., 1991, p. 227.

<u>Chapter Five</u>

1. 2 Chronicles 30:8-9, 17-22.

2. 2 Corinthians 7:10.

3. Chittister, Joan, D., OSB. <u>Life Ablaze: A Woman's Novena</u>. Erie, PA: *Benetvision*, 1997, p. 38. Citing, Julian of Norwich: "All shall be well. And all shall be well. And all manner of things shall be well."

4. Philippians 3:7-11.

<u>Chapter Six</u>

1. Webster, op. cit., p. 523.

2. Menninger, William C. [A bookmark.] Topeka, KS: The Menninger Clinic, 1996.

3. Pennington, M. Basil. <u>William of Saint Thierry: The Way to Divine Union</u>. Hyde Park, NY: New City Press, 1998, pp. 123-129.

4. Ibid., p. 124.

5. Ibid., p. 92.

6. Ibid.

7. Isaiah 26:3.

Chapter Seven

1.	Pennington, op. cit., p. 64.

2.	Delery, Father Mark. 2008. An observation made in an early reading of this manuscript. Father Mark is the author of The Parable of the Cherry Blossom. Berryville, VA: The Community of Cistercians of the Strict Observance, Inc., 1989. A glorious life-book. Thank you, Cousin Mark.

3.	Brouillet, Sara, D. From, "That You May Know God," a copyrighted poem, written in morning prayer on November 11, 2001, two months to the day, after 09/11/2001. In card form, the poem has been carried in the uniform breast pocket of American soldiers in the U.S. military conflict with Iraq.

4.	Gröning, Philip. *Into Great Silence.* 2005@ Philip Gröning Filmproduktion/Bavaria Film GmbH/ventura film sa/cine; 2007, Zeitgeist Films Ltd. An exquisite film, created over a six-month period in the grace-filled relationships between Philip Gröning and the monks of the Grande Chartreuse, who permitted and welcomed Philip into their lives and home in the French Alps. A stunning and life-changing work.

5.	Underhill, Evelyn. The School of Charity. Longman Group, UK, Limited, 1934. The edition, cited, of *The School of Charity* was first published by Morehouse Publishing by arrangement with Longman Group, UK, Limited, 1991, pp. 51-55.

6.	Ibid., p. 57.

7.	Fowler, James. From a discussion of Fowler's stages of faith development in a *science and religion* class, 1997. St. Mary's Seminary and University, Ecumenical Institute of Theology, Baltimore, MD.

Getting Back in the River

:an be ordered directly by completing this form and
enclosing a check made payable to:

=ather's Press, LLC
?424 SE 6th Street
_ee's Summit, MO 64063

=or $14.95*   *Quantity discounts available. Call Father's
                    Press, 816-600-6288 for details.

)eliver to:

Name_____

Street_____ Apt #_____

City_____ St_____ Zip_____

- OR -

?resent this information to your book store to assist
hem in their ordering process.

SBN: 978-0-9825321-3-3

ISBN: 978-0-9825321-3-3

51495

$14.95

9 780982 532133